# FITNESS
# CYCLING

## Shannon Sovndal, MD

Human Kinetics

## Library of Congress Cataloging-in-Publication Data

Sovndal, Shannon, 1970-
  Fitness cycling / Shannon Sovndal, MD.
     pages cm
  Includes index.
  1. Cycling. 2. Cycling--Equipment and supplies. I. Title.
  GV1041.S65 2013
  796.6--dc23

                              2012050503

ISBN-10: 1-4504-2930-0 (print)
ISBN-13: 978-1-4504-2930-6 (print)

Exercises in chapter 12 are adapted, by permission, from S. Sovndal, 2009, *Cycling Anatomy* (Champaign, IL: Human Kinetics), pp. 90, 92, 102, 104, 128, 130, 152, 154, 156, 170, and 174.

The web addresses cited in this text were current as of February 2013, unless otherwise noted.

**Acquisitions Editor:** Tom Heine; **Developmental Editor:** Bethany J. Bentley; **Assistant Editors:** Claire Marty and Elizabeth Evans; **Copyeditor:** Patrick Connolly; **Indexer:** Dan Connolly; **Permissions Manager:** Martha Gullo; **Graphic Designer:** Nancy Rasmus; **Graphic Artist:** Julie L. Denzer; **Cover Designer:** Keith Blomberg; **Photograph (cover):** Tim DeFrisco/Stellar Stock/age fotostock; **Photographs (interior):** pp. 1, 57 Tim DeFrisco/Stellar Stock/age footstock; p. 7 © Tom Bayer/fotolia; p. 21 Odilon Dimier/PhotoAlto/age footstock; p. 35 © Minik29 | Dreamstime.com; p. 47 © Bambi L. Dingman | Dreamstime.com; p. 71 © Doug James | Dreamstime.com; p. 87 © homydesign/fotolia; pp. 101, 115, 181, 193 Franck Faugere/DPPI/Icon SMI; p. 129 Corey Nolen/Aurora Photos; p. 145 © Maxim Petrichuk | Dreamstime.com; p. 165 Andreas Pollok/Cultura RM/age fotostock; **Photo Asset Manager:** Laura Fitch; **Visual Production Assistant:** Joyce Brumfield; **Photo Production Manager:** Jason Allen; **Art Manager:** Kelly Hendren; **Associate Art Manager:** Alan L. Wilborn; **Illustrations:** © Human Kinetics; **Printer:** Versa Press

We thank Streets Fitness in Louisville, CO, and Durst Cycle and Fitness in Urbana, IL, for assistance in providing the locations for the photo shoots for this book.

Human Kinetics books are available at special discounts for bulk purchase. Special editions or book excerpts can also be created to specification. For details, contact the Special Sales Manager at Human Kinetics.

Printed in the United States of America     10  9  8  7  6  5  4  3  2  1

The paper in this book is certified under a sustainable forestry program.

**Human Kinetics**
Website: www.HumanKinetics.com

*United States:* Human Kinetics
P.O. Box 5076
Champaign, IL 61825-5076
800-747-4457
e-mail: humank@hkusa.com

*Canada:* Human Kinetics
475 Devonshire Road Unit 100
Windsor, ON N8Y 2L5
800-465-7301 (in Canada only)
e-mail: info@hkcanada.com

*Europe:* Human Kinetics
107 Bradford Road
Stanningley
Leeds LS28 6AT, United Kingdom
+44 (0) 113 255 5665
e-mail: hk@hkeurope.com

*Australia:* Human Kinetics
57A Price Avenue
Lower Mitcham, South Australia 5062
08 8372 0999
e-mail: info@hkaustralia.com

*New Zealand:* Human Kinetics
P.O. Box 80
Torrens Park, South Australia 5062
0800 222 062
e-mail: info@hknewzealand.com

E5717

To the love of my life, Stephanie.
Thank you for inspiring me and everyone
around you. You're amazing.

# Contents

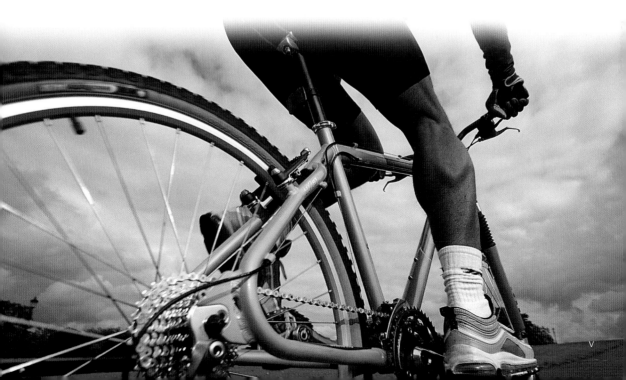

# Foreword

**Everyone** wants to ride their bike faster. Whether you are a professional cyclist working towards the Tour de France or simply looking to have more fun on weekend group rides, nothing is more satisfying than training hard and being rewarded with better performance. Approaching your training with a systematic approach supported by science is the key to realizing these performance breakthroughs. In *Fitness Cycling* Shannon Sovndal will provide you with the tools you need to train more effectively, climb stronger, sprint faster, and become a well-rounded cyclist.

I was drawn to the sport of cycling simply because I loved to ride my bike. The freedom of climbing onto a bicycle and taking off in whatever direction was intoxicating. Quickly I developed a hunger to become a better, faster cyclist. This desire drove me to seek knowledge about training and performance. The potential to maximize my performance through smarter training was astounding! Not only could I still experience the freedom of an open road, but I also discovered the pleasure in setting a goal, building a training program, and then executing my plan to achieve my objective. This formula, repeated throughout the years, allowed me to realize my dreams and become a professional cyclist, competing in the biggest events in the world.

I have worked with Shannon since 2009 as the team doctor for the professional cycling team Garmin-Sharp-Barracuda. Not only is he a great guy, but he has a skill for translating complex scientific principles of health and training into layman's terms. We have had many interesting conversations over the years that have opened my eyes to ways of riding my bike faster. He has helped me to come back from injuries quicker and stronger than before and helped me to understand just what is going on in my body as I work toward my goals. Shannon's medical background, years of competition as a cyclist, and hands-on experience working with world-class athletes give him a unique perspective of training and performance.

As with anything worthwhile, becoming a better cyclist requires hard work and commitment. But without a comprehensive plan to address both your strengths and your weaknesses, it is incredibly difficult to recognize your true potential. In this book, Shannon will help you to set goals and understand the necessary steps to get from where you are now to where you want to be.

Good luck and enjoy your training!

—Tyler Farrar

*Tyler Farrar is a member of Team Garmin-Sharp-Barracuda.*
*He has won stages in the Tour de France, Giro di Italia,*
*and Vuelta a Espana and is also an Olympian.*

# Preface

**Cycling** is a fantastic sport! Enjoying the outdoors, seeing the sights, experiencing the thrill of riding fast, and improving your fitness are all rolled up into a simple activity that most of us learned when we were children. *Fitness Cycling* is written to take you to the next level of your cycling and to help you get the most out of your time on the bike. If you've picked up this book, you've likely been out riding your bike and exploring the sport of cycling. But now you want more—more knowledge, more direction, and more motivation to really improve your riding technique, skills, and fitness. *Fitness Cycling* can help you do just that.

## Performance Rider

If you are time constrained, are tired of the same old ride, and want to get the most out of your time on the bike, then this book is perfect for you. Many cycling books approach fitness as if you're training for the Tour de France. In reality, most people have too many other commitments to solely focus on riding and training.

*Fitness Cycling* is written for the performance rider, an athlete who is interested in more than merely "going on a ride." This book is designed to take you from the basics of training to the details of creating your own training program. I understand that life is full of stresses and that numerous aspects are constantly pulling you every which way. That's why I wrote *Fitness Cycling*—to give you concise and focused direction in your training.

All cyclists should have goals for their riding. Goals keep you focused and give direction to your training. In this book, you'll learn how to use your riding to improve your fitness and reach your full potential as a rider. Whether your goal is besting a personal record up a hill climb, completing a century, or just improving your fitness, you will achieve remarkable results if you have a planned approach to your riding.

## Philosophy, Training Science, and Improving Your Performance

*Fitness Cycling* will provide you with a solid foundation in the sport of cycling. Although the primary focus of the book is providing focused workouts and training plans, it will also cover valuable information on bike equipment, proper position and fit, and training theory.

Training is more efficient and effective when you have a solid foundation in the science of training. *Fitness Cycling* will lay out the basic principles of training. It will also show you how to assess and track your fitness and training effort. Don't worry, my plan isn't to bore you to death with technical training information. I hope that the explanations are clear and concise and that the information will help you design your own training programs in the future.

## Workouts and Programs

The workout chapters are at the heart of the book. Each chapter covers a specific aspect of riding—base training, climbing, flatland threshold training, time trialing, and so on. The beginning of each workout chapter includes an explanation of the importance of that type of training and how it fits into a training program.

In each workout chapter, you will find detailed descriptions of 8 to 10 entertaining and effective training rides. Each workout includes specific cycling tips that will help you build your knowledge about riding, training, and cycling. Finally, sample workout programs are provided at the end of each chapter. My hope is that after you get through the book and use these programs, you'll be able to piece together a training program—mixing and matching the workouts provided—to create your own personalized training plan.

So, no more time to waste! Let's get started!

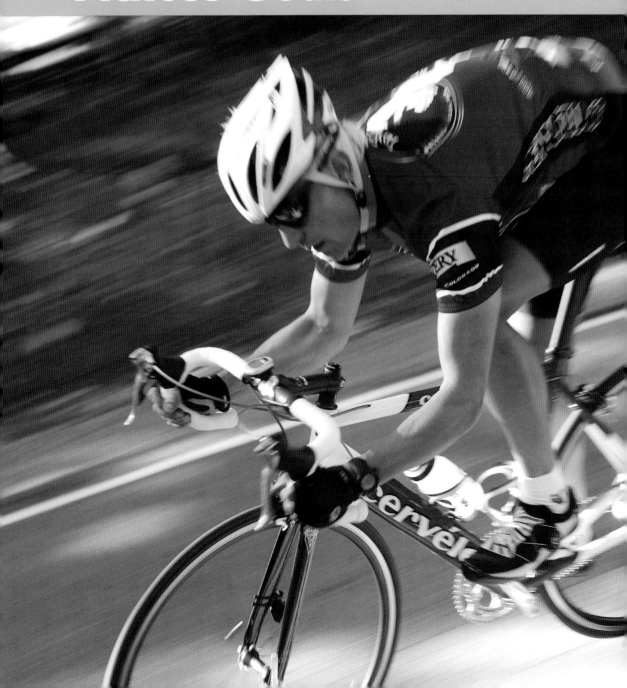

# Setting Cycling Fitness Goals

1

**For** many people, cycling is a passion. If you've cracked open this book, then you might feel the same way. Cycling is a phenomenal form of cardio-vascular exercise for people of all levels of fitness, age, and ability. It can provide a safe haven of solitude after a difficult workday, or it can serve as a social get-together that helps you bond with friends. You can push the limits of your perseverance and performance all from the solitude of your own brain. Cycling allows you to test yourself, to strive to be better, and to gauge your progression over time.

This book is all about helping you get the most out of your rides. It is written for the performance cyclist, for the rider who isn't satisfied with doing the same ride day after day. You may not have dreams (at least realistic ones) of winning the Tour de France, but you undoubtedly want to improve, build on your fitness, and test yourself and your ability on the bike.

Sport physiology and science can be a bit overwhelming. We've learned so much about training efficiently and effectively that the volume of information can become confusing. This book helps make that information understand-able and applicable to your daily riding. No matter what your goals are, you need to get the most out of every ride. That might simply mean having the most fun or going farther than ever before. Whatever you set out to do, you should do it with drive, passion, and a plan. Just because you're not paid to ride your bike doesn't mean that you can't apply the same types of systems that professionals use to reach their utmost potential.

## Training Goals

So, let's not waste any more time. If you want to train more seriously, you need to have a plan. Every time you get on your bike, you are essentially training. The question is whether you're training effectively or just gaining some conditioning through random episodes of exercise. If you are brand new to the sport, you will see great gains in your riding fitness, skill, and comfort simply by getting out on rides. Your body will respond to the stress of riding and will adapt accordingly. But, you can achieve much more pro-gression if you take the time to establish a plan of action.

Effective training is what this book is all about. Most of us have other commitments—family, work, friends, and so on. That's why cyclists need to make the most of the time they spend on the bike.

As a performance cyclist, you should always be striving to improve, and you should focus your attention on your cycling goals. If you want to hit the target, you first have to define that target.

What are your goals? Why are you riding your bike? Are you riding in order to stay healthy, to beat a friend up a local climb, or to complete your first century? Every person has a different goal, and that's the point. You own your goals and all the training that you complete—every pedal stroke, every climb, every Saturday you drag yourself out of bed and onto the road.

Goals can be intimidating because they come with an inherent chance of failure. A goal that is easy to achieve and includes no chance of failure would be ineffective because it goes against the very premise of this book—getting the most out of your riding. The possibility of success or failure is the crux of a good goal. You need to struggle to improve, and the only way to truly struggle is to know that there is a risk of failure. It is the risk, the chance of failure, that drives you toward success.

To help ensure that you establish attainable goals, you should apply the Four *Ps* of goal setting: personalized, positive, perceivable, and possible.

*Personalized* means that the goals are your own. Only you can determine what is important, what will motivate you to keep your commitment, and what will give you a sense of accomplishment.

All your goals should be *positive.* Negative energy sucks! At Disneyland, they live by this philosophy. If you ask the workers when the park closes, they will respond, "The park *stays open* until 8 o'clock." You should set a goal to accomplish a desired result rather than to avoid failure. Word your goals so that the outcome is positive.

You need to set goals that have a tangible outcome. Your goals must be *perceivable* to yourself or to others. This aspect of goal setting is all about accountability.

Finally, your goals need to be realistic but challenging. When you think about your goal, you should have a strong sense that the desired outcome is *possible,* but by no means assured. You need to believe even with the possibility of failure. This will help you suffer a little longer, struggle just a bit more, and get the most out of your training plan.

Don't think that goals are only for professionals or racers. EVERY RIDER NEEDS GOALS. Think of goals the same way you think of the rest of the training program. Training is all about progression, and goals should follow suit. They start with more obtainable outcomes. But with each accomplishment, the task becomes more difficult. Each goal builds on the last in a stepwise fashion (figure 1.1), until you find yourself faced with your ultimate accomplishment.

## Four *Ps* of Goal Setting

1. Personalized
2. Positive

3. Perceivable
4. Possible

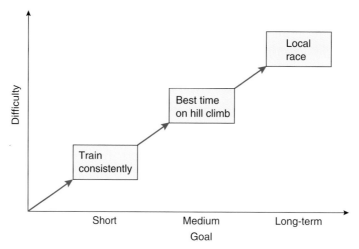

**Figure 1.1**  Goal progression.

Be sure to write down your goals. For each time frame—short, medium, and long—fill in your primary and secondary goals (figure 1.1). Again, these goals can be anything. They should be whatever motivates you to train when you might feel like flicking on the TV instead. There is something about actually writing down your goals. This brings them outside your brain and into the real world—an accountable world.

Training is all about commitment, discipline, and perseverance. It is a slow grind, and sometimes you feel as though you're going backward instead of forward. But if you stick to your program, you WILL get better. Writing down your goals is the first barrier to overcome.

Goals will perpetually be included in your training program. Every time you reach a goal, you can have a little celebration, even if it is internal. Treat yourself to a double half-caf, mocha chai latte if that's your thing. As soon as you are finished basking in the glory of the accomplishment, write down a new set of goals. Stay on target!

# RACE

My training philosophy includes four fundamental aspects that will help you reach your goals. *RACE* is a simple acronym that represents each of the key components: rest, accountability, consistency, and efficiency (figure 1.2).

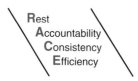

**Figure 1.2**  Key components for reaching your goals.

## Rest

In discussing a training philosophy, it may be odd to start by talking about rest, but that's exactly what I'm going to do. You don't get better while you're training. You get better while you're resting. Resting is where it all goes down; it's where you grow mitochondria, increase your vascularization, enhance your oxygen delivery—in other words, all the things that make you go faster on the bike.

Many athletes waste significant effort because they fail to give their body time to adapt to their training load. The purpose of your training is to stress your physiology, causing an alarm reaction and the subsequent adaptation. On a fundamental level, training damages your muscles. This damage needs time to heal, and the healing process is what takes you to the next level. Your fitness gains don't come while you're suffering on the bike during a hard training ride. They come after you've finished, when you take time to rest, sleep, and kick up your feet.

Chapter 2 will cover how your body adapts to training. If you train too much, your body can become exhausted. Another term for this is *overtraining*. As you train, each ride places a stress on your physiology. This stress results in adaptation, but the cost of the stress is fatigue. If you don't give your body enough rest, then the fatigue takes over and derails the entire train.

## Accountability

We all need accountability. It helps us stay true to our goals and our training plan. Self-accountability starts with you documenting your goals and your plan. Your master training plan lays out the course of action that will help you reach your goals. That's why you need to write down your goals and why you should keep a training diary. By documenting your performance day to day, you'll have a record of where you stand. You'll know the areas that you're excelling in and the areas where you're deficient. Don't be intimidated by documenting and reading over your faults. Use them to your advantage to revamp your training so you can reach your goals—even if it takes a bit longer than you originally anticipated.

If you have a spouse, a coach, or a good riding partner, let this person know about your goals. Fill the person in on how you hope to reach your goals and the basics of your training plan. This person can offer support and advice when you struggle or lose confidence. Also, when you know that someone besides yourself is aware of what you expect to accomplish, it add another level to your commitment.

## Consistency

Success is all about consistency. Conditioning requires commitment and sacrifice for a long period of time. Your fitness increases in baby steps, one step building on top of the other. But as soon as you take a break, or stop training, you start to move backward. This is called reversibility, or detraining. A difficult thing about training is that you lose your fitness faster than you gain it. So, the more time you spend not riding, the longer it will take to get back to your original level of fitness.

That's why being consistent is so important. We all have busy lives, and unless you make your living racing a bike, other things will have to take priority, regardless of how committed you are to riding. If you can predict your busy or stressful times, you can plan your training program to accommodate them. For example, a "rest" week might conveniently be planned during a big work project or a family vacation. If you unexpectedly have to take a break, try to limit your loss. Even a ride once a week can slow your deconditioning. Don't get down on yourself if your training takes a hit. It will at some point. That's just life. You need to focus on the long haul. You'll get your conditioning back over time. Just keep plugging away and try to limit your losses as much as possible.

## Efficiency

Every time you get on your bike, you should have a purpose. At first glance, this might sound a little extreme, but it will help you get the most out of your time on the bike. Rather than just "going on a ride," think about the reason why you're rolling out of the garage. Endurance, weight loss, speed, fun, and stress relief are all reasons why cyclists clip into the pedals and hit the road. If you consciously think about the purpose of the ride before, during, and after it, you'll find that your body responds. Focusing on the purpose enhances your training response. If you start to become bored or lose focus with your training program, change it up. You must stay fired up and excited about the bike.

It is easy to skim over this first chapter thinking that you'll get into the real meat of training in the later sections. That is the wrong approach! Setting goals before you begin is extremely important. The RACE acronym holds true for all levels of athletes, and if you are able to continually think about each aspect—rest, accountability, consistency, and efficiency—you'll find that your training brings you to new heights.

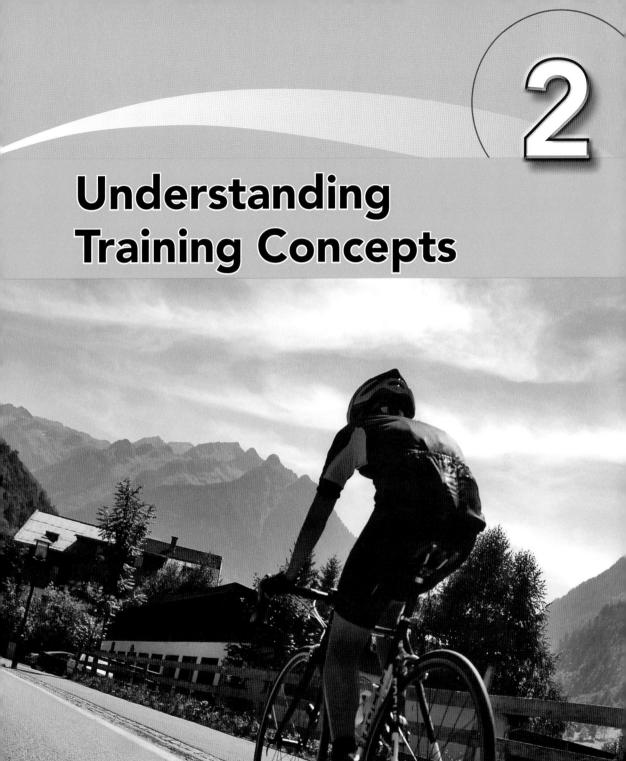

# Understanding Training Concepts

**2**

# Cyclists

**Cyclists** train to improve their endurance and to become faster and stronger. Each physiologic system is stressed by the imposed workload, and over time, the cyclist tries to get the amount of training just right, bringing about better performance.

Economics teaches the fundamental principles of supply, demand, and scarcity. These drive the rise and fall of businesses, industries, and even countries. These same principles are also fundamental to the performance cyclist. Athletes use energy supplied from their cardiovascular system to power their musculoskeletal system. To simplify, this energy comes from a combination of calories and oxygen, and as an athlete increases his intensity, the supply cannot always keep up with the demand. Energy becomes scarce, and the athlete's physiologic system becomes limited in its capacity to do work.

That is why athletes train. The Olympic motto is "Citius, Altius, Fortius"—which means swifter, higher, stronger! To reach the next level, you need to understand a few points that will guide your training program. A physiology lesson is beyond the scope of this book, but this chapter covers some broad concepts to help you gain a general understanding of the reasoning behind your workouts and training program.

## Adaptation

Obviously, training makes you better. But why? The answer is adaptation. The human body resists change. Like Newton's first law, a body at rest tends to stay at rest. Your body wants the status quo. In physiology, this is called homeostasis.

On a fundamental level, your body's innate desire is to remain stable and unstressed. Training messes this all up. When you work out, you place a new stressor on your system. The alarm bells sound, and homeostasis is disturbed. As a result, your body tries to mitigate any future experience with this stress. It adapts to the workout and therefore better tolerates the increased demands in the future. This all takes time, and your training program is built around the concept of stress and rest, leading to the resultant adaptation.

Figure 2.1 shows how your body responds to a training stress. Immediately after the stress, your body is fatigued. But slowly, your body adapts, and your fitness jumps to a higher level. If you did the same workout again, your body would be ready, there wouldn't be any real fatigue, and you would stay at the new higher level.

You need to keep a couple of key points in mind. The first is that you can't always do the same workout. If you do, your body will eventually have no

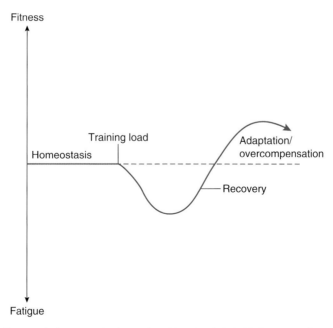

**Figure 2.1** Fitness, fatigue, and adaptation. Your body is initially at rest (homeostasis) until you apply a training load. This results in fatigue followed by recovery. It doesn't stop there, however. To resist the stress in the future, your body adapts, or overcompensates. The result is an increased level of fitness.

alarm reaction, and you will get no adaptation. Perhaps you have experience going to the gym and doing the same workout over and over. If so, you likely saw no real change in your fitness or physique. This is because, over time, the workout doesn't cause any stress. You plateau because your body has adapted to the workout and established a new status quo. That is why you always need to change and progress your workouts.

The second point is that you need to give your body time to adapt. You need to rest. Chapter 1 explained my training philosophy based on the RACE acronym. Rest was the first point addressed. Don't overdo your training. Remember, the adaptation doesn't occur during the workout. It happens AFTER the workout. If you continually apply too much stress, your body can become exhausted and overtrained.

This concept is referred to as the general adaptation syndrome (GAS), which includes three components:

1. Alarm reaction
2. Adaptation
3. Exhaustion

Ideally, as you train, your body keeps bouncing back and forth between phases 1 and 2, alarm reaction and adaptation. This will move you to an ever higher level of fitness and performance. Only when you overdo it—when you make a mistake in your training stress—do you move to the exhaustion phase.

Think of training load stimulus as the flame of a campfire. As you slowly apply the stimulus, your marshmallow responds by becoming soft, brown, and delicious. If you apply too much heat or flame, the marshmallow begins to burn and char (figure 2.2). The same is true with your training. The perfect amount of load brings about the desired response. Too much training load and you'll become overheated and overworked.

The best way to avoid overtraining is to listen to your body. It is normal to feel fatigued during a particular cycle of your training program (this is often planned). But, if your fatigue starts to move to the next level, then it's time to back off and allow yourself some good recovery time. This could be a couple of days or even a week. Keeping a training diary (see chapter 5) will help you monitor your training and fatigue. A training diary is an invaluable tool for keeping track of exactly where you stand in relation to training load and fatigue. You will be able to look back over your past training cycles to see how you've performed on well-known or repeated rides. Has your performance been dropping off? Have you been more fatigued than in the past? Do the rides seem much more difficult than they used to?

In a good training program, the athlete is always balancing stress, fatigue, and recovery. As I've said before, true adaptation occurs while resting, not while training. Be sure to always give yourself adequate recovery time after a training load. This will vary based on the load, so always listen to your

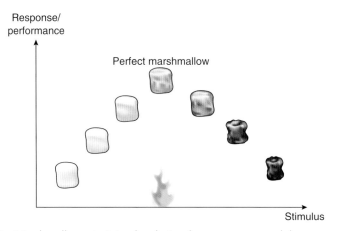

**Figure 2.2**  Marshmallows: training load stimulus–response model.

Based on an illustration by Dr. Allen Lim.

## Overtraining

Here are some warning signs that you may be overtraining or exhausted:

- Continued poor performance on the bike
- Poor sleep
- Ongoing muscle aches or frequent cramping
- Elevated heart rate in the morning or on a routine ride
- Agitation and poor motivation

body. Any time you enter the exhaustion phase, you've either given yourself too much stress, not enough recovery, or both. To train smartly, you need to constantly tweak your training program based on your perceived level of fitness and fatigue.

## Progression

Training fundamentally strives for progression. Each training day brings something new and builds on all that you've done previously. Each effort is part of the overall plan. Like building a Lego structure, the layers are laid down one before the next until the structure grows higher and higher. Your training program is similar to building a staircase; each new step brings you closer to your overall goal.

Following the GAS model, you'll apply stress with each workout and then wait for the adaptation. As time goes on, you'll continue bouncing between alarm reaction and adaptation. The cool part is that slowly you'll be able to apply more and more stress with each workout. If you look at your training diary, you'll see that your body is becoming stronger and fitter. You'll continually move up to the next platform, which will be your new step-off point.

Note that progression should involve a methodical approach. Slow, progressive steps result in the most long-term gains. This is also the best way to strengthen your core and avoid injuries. You should avoid being a weekend warrior—that is, you should avoid trying to do a maximal-load workout without laying the foundation. You can't make up a week or month's worth of work in a day just because you suddenly have time or feel guilty. Progress takes patience. Think *slow and steady*. Progression requires each layer to be laid on the previous foundation (figure 2.3). This takes commitment and time, but ultimately it will help you reach your peak fitness and performance.

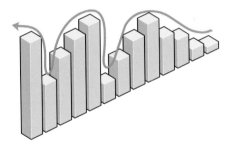

**Figure 2.3** Progression is a stair-step model.

# Specificity

Every sport requires a unique set of qualities. Obviously, an Olympic heavy-weight powerlifter won't make the best Giro d'Italia racer, and bike riders usually make poor powerlifters. You need to train for your sport. Although there is some crossover between different endurance activities, you must train specifically on the bike if you want to focus your work and improve your performance. There's no substitute for time in the saddle if you want to be the best rider possible. Adaptation comes as a result of stress, and the changes in your physiology are specific to your sport and to the alarm reaction brought on by training.

To be good at anything, you have to practice specifically in that field. There is no substitute, and there is no way around it. Every time you ride, you're working on your form, cadence, position, and fitness. You're adapting to your specific sport.

Many cyclists cross-train in the off-season, and this can be an effective addition to your training. Participation in other sports can complement your cycling performance, but only to a degree. If you have limited time and you are committed to your bike, then the majority of your workouts should be spent riding. That's the simple truth of specificity. There's no surrogate for the real thing!

# Individuality

Each person is unique—in life and in sport. Remember that what might work for one athlete may not be best for another. Every person responds differently to a given workload. Many factors—including your physiology, your level of fatigue, and your outside life stressors—must be taken into account. You must cater your training to only one person: you! We all respond to stress differently, and we all have different performance capabilities. That is what makes a good training program so challenging and fun.

Even for top athletes, it's difficult to perfectly gauge how a given stress will result in a desired adaptation. Every year, riders try to peak for the Tour de France. But getting the timing just right—getting your engine to work maximally during three weeks in July—is definitely a challenge, even for the most knowledgeable and seasoned professional. That is why athletes may have a good race one year and a lesser race another year.

Only you will truly know how a workout affects you. You need to get in tune with your senses. Listen to what your body tells you after a workout. Developing the ability to do this takes time and only comes with practice. Again, a good training diary will help you start to figure out how your body responds to various workloads and training stressors.

The workout programs in this book are meant as a starting point. Over time, you should start to tweak the workouts to best suit your own individual physiology. A good training program should be different for each person, molded perfectly to the strengths and weaknesses of each rider.

# Energy

Think of your body—and specifically, the musculoskeletal system—as an engine that requires fuel. Your diet, including everything you eat, makes up the energy source burned as fuel. Carbohydrate, fat, and protein all contribute to supplying the needed energy for your body to do work. Few things are clear-cut in human physiology, and choosing fuel sources based on intensity is no exception. That being said, to make nutrition sense on a practical level, you can assume that carbohydrate is the most efficient fuel for moderate- to higher-intensity workouts. Fat (and a bit of protein) is the primary source of fuel during low-intensity efforts. That is why workout machines in the gym are often labeled with signs that say Fat Burning Zone or Carbohydrate Burning Zone based on intensity level. (See the section Cycling for Weight Loss.)

Your body has a limited supply of carbohydrate (stored as glycogen) to burn during exercise. You'll get 1 to 2 hours of work before you burn up your stored supply. Fat, on the other hand (much to most people's chagrin), is abundant. But that is not necessarily a bad thing. A person needs an efficient, dense fuel source that can provide hours and hours of energy reserves, and fat does just that.

Regardless of whether you are burning carbohydrate, fat, or protein, the fuel is converted to the common energy currency used by the body—adenosine triphosphate (ATP). ATP supplies energy for basic cellular processes all the way to heavy-duty muscle work done while riding your bike. Unfortunately, ATP is not easily stored in the body, and for the most part, it is created on an as-needed basis.

Two types of metabolism occur in muscle cells during exercise. One produces energy relatively slowly (slow metabolism) and requires oxygen (aerobic). The other produces energy relatively quickly (fast metabolism) and does not require oxygen (anaerobic). However, this does not mean that the absence or presence of oxygen controls these energy pathways. Rather, both systems are always in play and working to create fuel for your muscles. But because each pathway produces energy at different rates, as your effort changes, the ratio of energy supplied by each type of metabolism also changes. You *preferentially* use one system over the other. When you're cruising on a ride at low to moderate effort, the majority of your energy comes from aerobic or slow metabolism. For short, high-energy efforts, most energy comes from anaerobic or fast metabolism.

During aerobic metabolism, the cardiovascular system oxygenates blood in the lungs and pumps it throughout the body, supplying oxygen for the creation of the ATP. This generally occurs at lower intensities before the demand outstrips the oxygen supply.

Anaerobic metabolism, or ATP creation without oxygen, occurs in two different physiologic systems—the phosphate system and the glycolysis system. The phosphate system supplies energy for roughly 10 seconds of full effort before depletion. The glycolysis system has a bit more staying power but not much when compared with the aerobic system. The glycolysis system can anaerobically make ATP for only a few minutes. It produces high energy at a high cost, and you'll definitely feel the effort soon after starting. You can only rely on this for so long before the burn, pain, and breathing rate force you to decrease your effort.

You may be wondering where lactic acid comes into all of this. Historically, lactic acid has been used to quantify anaerobic metabolism, specifically glycolysis. However, new science has shed some light on the field, and this will be covered in chapter 3.

# Nutrition

If you are serious about your training and riding performance, then you must also be serious about your diet. Eating healthily ensures that your body will have optimal energy and nutrients during training and recovery.

Healthy living and athletic performance go hand in hand. Nutrition can be confusing, and sensationalized diet plans don't make things any easier. This book is by no means focused on nutrition, so if you have a lot of questions, you may want to pick up a sport nutrition book or meet with a certified nutritionist.

The previous section covered energy and fuel. You are what you eat, so make sure you're taking in high-quality food. Think of your body as a high-end sports car. Don't put low-grade unleaded fuel in your Ferrari!

Your diet—including carbohydrate, fat, and protein—will be used to make the energy nuggets discussed earlier. Part of a good diet plan is balancing your calorie intake from each food group with your expenditure. Dr. Matthew Rabin, a friend and colleague of mine, has provided some guidelines on proper nutrition for riding (see sidebar). Dr. Rabin is a chiropractor and nutrition guru whom I've worked with at Slipstream Sports.

## Proper Nutrition for Riding

by Matthew Rabin, DC, ICSSD

When you are training and racing, your nutritional approach is of the utmost importance. To begin to understand nutrition, you must first be aware of the basic fuel principles.

Food is fuel, and this fuel is broken down into carbohydrate, fat, and protein. We will focus on carbohydrate, because this is the fuel that your body uses most in endurance exercise.

Your daily carbohydrate input should be based on your specific training needs. Carbohydrate intake needs to be considered at three distinct times: before, during, and after your ride. The following information gives you the basics regarding the amount to consume if your training is of moderate intensity. Current approaches to nutrition have moved away from using percent as a way to measure food intake because it is difficult to grasp and does not provide enough detail. By adopting the following principles, you will quickly see the benefits as well as how simple they are to apply.

### Daily Intake of Carbohydrate

Consume approximately 5 to 7 grams of carbohydrate per kilogram of body weight. This will help ensure that your muscle glycogen stores are optimally maintained. The carbohydrate intake should be divided over your typical daily meal plan. For example, if you weigh 70 kilograms, you should consume between 350 and 490 grams of carbohydrate over the course of the day.

To be more specific, the timing of your carbohydrate intake can be broken down as follows:

### *Pre-Ride*

The timing of when you eat is important, especially when you are planning a hard session. You want to make sure that you are prepared and have the sustained energy (called carbohydrate availability) for the upcoming session.

Before a hard session, you should consume about 1 to 3 grams per kilogram of body weight during the period from 1 to 4 hours before exercise.

> continued

> *continued*

### During the Ride

If you are riding for a period of up to an hour, you should not need to consume food on the bike. If you are riding for over an hour of moderate to intense exercise, then taking in between 30 and 60 grams of carbohydrate per hour will keep your energy stores sustained. The body can adequately digest this amount, but you should practice eating on the bike to see what foods you can tolerate while riding. Sport foods and gels offer a great way to eat on the bike and also easily calculate the carbohydrate intake.

### Post-Ride

When you return from your ride, you have a small window of opportunity to optimally replenish muscle glycogen stores. These days the experts recommend that you consume your recovery meal within 45 minutes of the end of the ride.

Taking in 1 gram of carbohydrate per kilogram of body weight will provide you with the optimal amount of fuel for recovery. Also note that taking in 20 grams of lean protein will further aid your recovery.

© Matthew Rabin. Used with permission.

For all your nutritional needs, you can get what you need from food and meals. However, with the number of sport foods, gels, and bars on the market these days, you can easily find additional sources to help you target the right amount of carbohydrate at the right time around your ride. Have fun and be creative with your food choices. Keep the previous principles in mind while determining the proper foods for your training routine.

As a general rule, you should try to eat "from the edges of the grocery store." This is where you'll find fresh produce and unprocessed foods. Lean meat, fish, unsaturated fat, and complex carbohydrate (such as whole grains and brown rice) give you the energy, fiber, vitamins, and minerals that your body needs to train efficiently. Here are a few key points that can help guide your diet plan:

- Base meal choices on nutrient-dense foods: fruits, vegetables, lean protein, whole grains, and essential fats.
- Avoid overly refined and processed foods.
- Avoid dead calories: soft drinks, alcohol, fast food.
- Spread your meals out over the course of the day. Numerous small meals are better than one or two huge meals.

Carbohydrate has received a lot of press in the last few years. Specifically, numerous diet plans have regarded carbohydrate as "bad." However, remember that carbohydrate (and glycogen, which is the storage form of carbohydrate) acts as your muscle's major fuel source during prolonged physical activity. Your goal is optimal performance while training, not a quick scheme to cause the numbers on a scale to drop a few notches. If you are training heavily, you'll need to include carbohydrate in your diet. Some carbohydrate choices are better than others. Here is a list of good and bad sources of carbohydrate:

**Good:**
- Fruits
- Vegetables
- Beans
- Legumes
- Nuts
- Whole-grain breads, cereals, and pasta

**Bad:**
- Refined grains (white bread, white rice)
- Processed foods (cakes, cookies, chips)
- Soft drinks
- Candy bars
- Alcohol

# Cycling for Weight Loss

Cycling is a fantastic way to lose weight. Regardless of what a trendy diet might try to tell you, an effective weight loss program includes two key aspects: (1) exercise and (2) eating right. For you to lose weight over time, the calories you take in or eat must be less than the calories you burn. It's a simple solution to what seems like a complex problem:

Weight Loss = Calories In < Calories Out

That might seem like work, and it is! Losing weight is tough. You'll need to follow the same principles that are applied to training. Be consistent and persistent. Changing your base weight is like turning a ship with a small rudder. It takes a little while for the ship to respond to a change of direction. The change will come; you just have to be patient.

Some cyclists make the mistake of only wanting to ride in the "fat burning zone." The reality of weight loss is that you need to burn calories. The harder you ride, the faster you'll burn. This extrapolates beyond the workout as well. So if you only have a limited amount of time and want to get the most weight loss out of your workout, you should ride as fast as you can.

Going out on a ride is one of the best ways to burn calories. But burning calories is not all that cycling offers. It can help you lower blood pressure, build muscle, and improve cardiovascular health—all while rekindling the childhood thrill of zipping down the road with the wind blowing in your face.

Cycling offers a wide range of gradable training intensities, allowing you to find your perfect training tempo. You can train indoors and out. And cycling is easy on your muscles, joints, and tendons. It's a great way to get yourself back into shape if you've been out of the workout game for a while.

Cycling's weight loss benefits include the following:

- Use of large muscle groups to burn calories
- Easily varied intensities
- Low-impact, non-weight-bearing exercise
- Aerobic, resistance, and isometric exercises all in one workout
- Fresh air, beautiful scenery, and socializing with riding partners
- Effective exercise for all ages

# Hydration

Hydration is key to your success. You can train perfectly the entire off-season and approach your goal in peak form, but if you let yourself become dehydrated, you could see all your hard work go down the drain. It may seem like a simple task, but avoiding dehydration can be tricky. Losing even 1 percent of your body weight to dehydration can have notable changes in your performance. Losses of 2 to 4 percent are even more pronounced and cause marked changes in your cardiovascular system and thermoregulation.

Athletes have high variability in their sweating rate and in the concentration of sodium in their perspiration. On a cool day, some athletes will sweat as little as 200 milliliters per hour, while on a hot day, some can produce more than 2 liters of sweat per hour. Sodium loss in sweat is highly variable, ranging from 400 to 1,200 milligrams per liter. Imagine if you have a prolonged workout, losing over 5 liters of sweat. That could be close to 6,000 milligrams of sodium lost just by training! Looking over these figures, it quickly becomes apparent that keeping up with sweat and sodium loss can be a considerable task.

Because of the wide variability in sweating rates, there is no simple formula or solution for keeping a cyclist well hydrated. Some generalizations can be made, however. It is better to be overhydrated than underhydrated, and if you are taking in the proper mix of fluid and electrolytes, you don't have to worry about some of the downside of overhydration with plain water (hyponatremia). No matter how hard you train or how fit you become, if you fail to simply rehydrate during your workout, much of your preparatory effort will be lost to inefficiency and underperformance.

Hydration should become second nature. You should develop an internal clock that prompts you to grab your water bottle and take a swig. A good general rule is to take a drink every 15 minutes. Aim to empty your bottle every hour. If the temperature is hot or you are riding hard, increase this to two bottles per hour. During big stage races such as the Tour de France and Giro d'Italia, riders frequently go through three or four bottles per hour (sometimes even more). If you get behind in your hydration, it's tough to catch up, so your best option is to stay ahead of the hydration game.

Before, during, and after training, you should drink fluid that replaces what you're using up; this includes sugar, sodium, potassium, magnesium, and calcium, to name a few. Many commercial drinks are available that will do the trick. Some are more palatable than others, especially when you're working hard, so you should try them out to see which one suits you best. Skratch Labs has created a scientifically made formula that works extremely well for replacing fluids and electrolytes when a person is performing hard-effort exercise. The product is called Exercise Hydration from Skratch. It was created by an excellent physiologist and close friend of mine, Dr. Allen Lim. See the Hyponatremia sidebar.

A simple way to monitor hydration status is with weight. A pre- and post-ride weight will give you a good idea of how much body fluid has been lost through the effort. Another straightforward monitoring method is to pay attention to the color of your urine and how frequently you urinate. If your output starts to drop off, this indicates that your body is hoarding the limited

## Hyponatremia

by Dr. Allen Lim

Your sweat contains both water and electrolytes like sodium, potassium, magnesium, calcium and chloride. Of these electrolytes, sodium is the most critical to normal bodily function. A decrease in your body's sodium concentration can lead to a number of problems ranging from a drop in performance, nausea, headache, confusion, irritability, vomiting, fatigue, muscle spasms, seizures, coma, and even death in very rare cases. A low sodium concentration in the blood is called Hyponatremia and can occur when a person who is sweating heavily drinks only water. Because sweat contains both water and sodium, replacing just the water and not the sodium can dilute the sodium in the body.

Sports drinks are designed to replace the sodium lost in sweat, but most contain too much sugar and not enough sodium. While the sodium lost in sweat can average 200 to 500 mg per half liter (16.9 oz), the sodium content in most sports drinks is only about 50 to 200 mg per half liter. Thus, it's important to look for a sports drink with at least 300 mg of sodium and no more than about 20 grams of sugar per half liter and to realize that these drinks are designed to be used when exercising, not when sitting around watching television. Finally, if you can't find a sports drink with enough sodium, make sure that you get plenty of salt in the food that you do eat during exercise.

supply of water that it has. If you note that your urine takes on a darker color, this may mean that it is becoming more concentrated. Remember that vitamin supplements can also darken your urine.

Keep in mind that thirst is a late indicator of hydration. If you're feeling thirsty, you've already dropped the ball. The importance of drinking early and often cannot be emphasized enough. Don't wait for your training partner or friend to drink. Be the first to grab a bottle and take a drink. It is a simple solution to a performance-ruining problem.

This chapter provided some broad and general concepts to help guide your training. Your goal is to use the "perfect" training load so that you can adapt and progress. Try not to overcook yourself. Because you want to be your best on the bike, you'll need to spend the majority of your time actually riding your bike. You need to take into account your own individuality and then tailor your training to meet your needs. Don't just blindly follow the plan of a riding friend. Finally, you need to pay attention to your diet and hydration. These are fundamental to efficient physiologic operation and energy supply. Keep all these concepts tucked in the back of your brain as you move on to the next chapter. Good fuel will provide energy to help you reach your full potential.

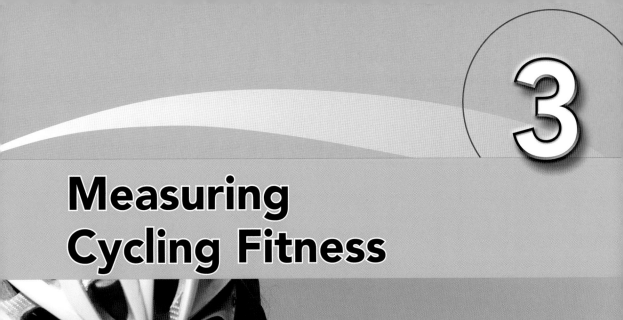

# Measuring Cycling Fitness

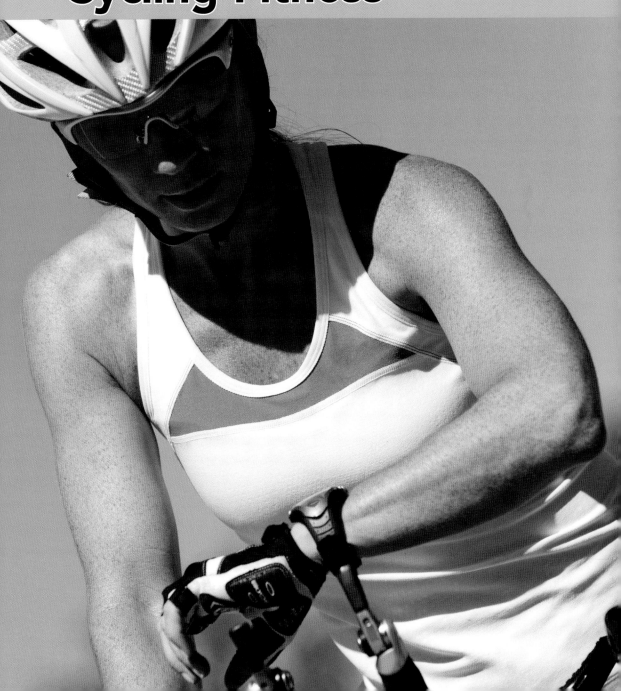

# 3

**You're** likely reading this book because you want to improve your cycling performance. Riding fast and with endurance is a matter of desire, natural ability, and an intelligent training program. Smart training relies on making the most of your time on the bike, and training efficiently means that you plan out your training rides based on your current fitness and your ultimate goal. So, how do you know your fitness level? What is your natural ability or potential? How do you train to enhance your inherent physiologic capabilities? Let's jump into the deep end and clear up the murky water.

Training is all about making your engine reach its optimal potential. As you train, two things happen. The first is that your motor "gets bigger." It is able to put out more horsepower. The second is that your motor becomes more efficient; you get more horsepower and less waste for a given amount of fuel. This is the reason why people spend so much time on their training programs. Sure, some people (e.g., Taylor Phinney or Tyler Farrar) are gifted with a V12 high-performance Ferrari engine, but the rest of us are working with a more common and cost-friendly model such as a Civic. Both the Ferrari engine and the Civic engine work essentially the same way, so regardless of your baseline physiology and particular engine model, training (and the resultant adaptation) can tune you up to your optimal potential.

This chapter will help you understand and assess your level of fitness and your potential. The chapter begins with an explanation of *maximal performance* ($\dot{V}O_2$max, maximal heart rate, and maximal power) and then gets into the concepts of *sustained performance* (lactate threshold heart rate and lactate threshold power). After you have a good understanding of how to determine and measure where you stand, you can begin to get into the fun stuff—actual training!

## Maximal Performance

Let's start with your $\dot{V}O_2$max. Maximal oxygen consumption ($\dot{V}O_2$max) is the maximal amount of oxygen that can be used by your body for maximal sustained power output. Based on your physiology, there is a maximal amount of oxygen that can be supplied by your lungs and transported by your cardiovascular system. This is the supply side of the equation. There is also a maximal capacity of oxygen that your muscles and tissue can use at any given moment. This is the demand side. Either side—supply or demand—can limit your maximal oxygen use. For most athletes, the limiting factor is supply.

Don't get lost in the details. Stay focused on the general principles. During exercise, the air you breathe supplies oxygen to your muscle cells. The mitochondria in these cells create ATP, which is used to power your muscles. More oxygen leads to more energy, and this results in more power, speed, and performance.

We'd all like to have a high $\dot{V}O_2$max. But the reality is that $\dot{V}O_2$max is largely (but not completely) determined by your genetics. There are only a few Greg LeMonds and Eddy Merckxs of the world. Maybe both of your parents were amazing endurance athletes, but if they weren't, you still have hope. First, $\dot{V}O_2$ is only part of the puzzle that makes up a great cyclist. Sure, you would need to have a certain baseline $\dot{V}O_2$ in order to race professionally, but that is not the goal of most cyclists. And with smart preparation, you can maximize your natural ability. Lactate threshold, appropriate peaking, nutrition, and tactics all come into play when you are trying to reach your goal.

Even though genetics has a big role, you can still move your $\dot{V}O_2$ to the next level. Training *can* make a difference. Some athletes are "responders" to $\dot{V}O_2$ training, meaning that they make big gains in their $\dot{V}O_2$max with training. However, even "nonresponders" will have an upward change in their $\dot{V}O_2$max with a good periodization training program.

True $\dot{V}O_2$max is a laboratory measurement, but even if you never plan on being a test subject yourself, gaining a good understanding of how $\dot{V}O_2$max is determined will help you train effectively. Let's take a look at the testing process.

In the laboratory, an athlete performs a graded exercise test (in this case, on a bike) while hooked up to a breathing apparatus and a computer (figure 3.1). In this setup, the athlete looks like a bicyclist on a trainer wearing a

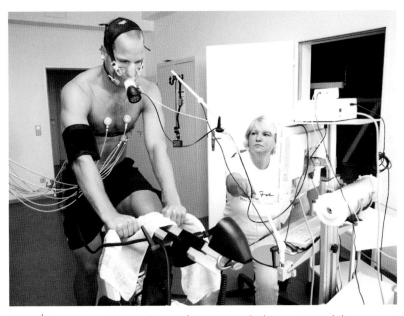

**Figure 3.1** $\dot{V}O_2$max test. The cyclist performs a graded stress test while a computer calculates oxygen consumption. The maximal amount of oxygen consumption is the athlete's "ceiling" or $\dot{V}O_2$max.

SCUBA regulator. The athlete incrementally performs more and more work at regular time intervals until the effort is too much and the "engine blows." The athlete can no longer keep the pace and must slow down.

For any sadists out there, you'll love watching someone suffer through one of these tests. The test takes an innocent athlete and slowly dials in the pain. The once happy-go-lucky cyclist becomes a grimacing, nauseated, air-sucking maniac. But that's the whole idea—to see how much air, and hence oxygen, the rider can pull into his lungs at his maximal effort.

By performing a calculation based on inspired and expired air, the computer system calculates the total amount of oxygen used by the body. If you like math, you can look over the Fick equation in figure 3.2. If math gives you bad dreams and an odd sense of anxiety, then just skip to the next paragraph.

Oxygen consumption increases linearly with exercise effort until the body reaches its maximal workload. At that point, no more oxygen can be consumed by your body's machinery. The oxygen consumption plateaus and ultimately drops off in the opposite direction because you are forced to reduce intensity .

$\dot{V}O_2$max is expressed in one of two ways. The first, absolute $\dot{V}O_2$max (liters of oxygen per minute), ranges from 3.0 to 6.0 for males and 2.5 to 5.0 for females. The second expression, called relative $\dot{V}O_2$max (milliliters of oxygen per kilogram of body weight per minute), falls between 26 and 96 ml/kg/min. Remember your science classes? The units of measurement are always important. Notice that the relative $\dot{V}O_2$max takes into account your

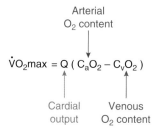

$$\dot{V}O_2\text{max} = Q\,(\,C_aO_2 - C_vO_2\,)$$

Arterial $O_2$ content

Cardial output

Venous $O_2$ content

**Figure 3.2**   The Fick equation.

## Putting $\dot{V}O_2$max in Perspective

- *Best male: 96 ml/kg/min*
- *Best female: 78.6 ml/kg/min*
- *Thoroughbred racehorse: 200 ml/kg/min*
- *Sled dog: 300 ml/kg/min*

body weight, whereas the absolute $\dot{V}O_2$max does not. An athlete will have vastly different looking numbers for these two measurements.

Table 3.1 will help you determine where you stand. The average untrained male will have a $\dot{V}O_2$max of roughly 45 ml/kg/min (3.5 L/min); an average untrained female will have a $\dot{V}O_2$max of 38 ml/kg/min (2.0 L/min). A well-trained collegiate cyclist may have a $\dot{V}O_2$max of 70 ml/kg/min. Greg LeMond is reported to have a $\dot{V}O_2$max of 92.5 ml/kg/min. Bjorn Daehlie, one of the great cross-country skiers from Norway, had a reported measurement of 96 ml/kg/min.

Perhaps you've already come to a simple conclusion regarding how to increase your relative $\dot{V}O_2$max. Lose a few pounds, and suddenly you've increased your performance ceiling! (You'll just have to make sure you use relative $\dot{V}O_2$max instead of absolute $\dot{V}O_2$max.)

### Table 3.1   $\dot{V}O_2$max: How Do You Measure Up?

| | Maximal oxygen uptake | | | |
| | Male | | Female | |
| Age | Excellent | Average | Excellent | Average |
| --- | --- | --- | --- | --- |
| 20-25 | >60 | 42-47 | >56 | 38-41 |
| 26-35 | >55 | 40-42 | >52 | 35-38 |
| 36-45 | >51 | 35-38 | >45 | 31-33 |
| 46-55 | >45 | 32-35 | >40 | 28-30 |
| 56+ | >41 | 30-32 | >37 | 25-27 |

## Maximal Heart Rate

So, how can you relate $\dot{V}O_2$max to your training? Well, the number itself doesn't do you much good. Professional teams can use it as a screening test to see if a cyclist has the fundamental ability to compete at the pro level, but cyclists don't routinely monitor how many liters of oxygen per minute their lungs are consuming while out on the bike. For the performance cyclist, gaining an understanding of the physiology behind $\dot{V}O_2$max helps you understand why maximal heart rate is an effective and practical alternative.

While $\dot{V}O_2$max directly measures your performance ceiling, maximal heart rate is an indirect measure, or an estimation, of your ceiling. Some equations can be used to make an approximation of $\dot{V}O_2$max based on an athlete's resting and maximal heart rates. But for practical purposes, because $\dot{V}O_2$ monitoring on the road is difficult, maximal heart rate (MHR) is a good substitute. Although some physiologists will argue the point, MHR is a poor man's way to measure and monitor your $\dot{V}O_2$max. MHR can help you guesstimate your ceiling. It also gives you a simple measurement that you can perform at home to monitor your progress and form.

In chapter 4, you will learn how to base your training on a percentage of your maximal heart rate. But first, you'll have to go through the steps of actually determining your own personal numbers. Figure 3.3 shows you how to find your MHR. The first method involves using a formula to calculate the MHR; the second method involves finding your MHR while you are riding your bike on the road.

## Maximal Power

If you have access to a power meter, you can use your maximal power to help guide and track your training. Some references base training intensity on a percentage of your maximal power.

Power meters were first used by professionals in the 1980s. Because of decreased cost and increased reliability, power meters have become much more common. These devices measure the torque either at the crank, bottom bracket, or rear hub. They are a useful training tool because they give a direct measurement of performance—of what you are actually doing on the bike. This is quite different than heart rate monitors, which make an indirect assessment of your performance. It's the difference between measuring the temperature of a car engine and measuring the torque produced by the driveshaft.

Don't worry if you don't have a power meter. A power meter is an expensive piece of equipment. Professionals use every bit of information they can: heart rate monitor, power meter, and perceived exertion (discussed in chapter 4). But training progress can be tracked by using any of these monitors individually or in combination.

Although understanding maximal heart rate and maximal power is important, the best method is to base your training on *sustained performance measurements*, which will be discussed in the next section.

Figure 3.4 presents the steps for finding your maximal power. You might be thinking that you can do the maximal heart rate and maximal power test at the same time, but this isn't necessarily the case. To find your maximal heart rate, you'll need more time to ramp up your heart. To find your maximal power, you only need to perform a maximal sprint. This can be done either on the flats or in the hills, but you should avoid a steep grade because you won't be able to maintain your leg speed (cadence) for a good measurement.

## Figure 3.3  Finding Your Maximal Heart Rate

**Calculated Method:**

Numerous formulas are used to calculate a person's maximal heart rate (MHR) based on age. Obviously, there can be a wide range of MHRs among individuals of the same age, so the formula method only provides a rough approximation. Here is the simplest and most common equation:

$$MHR = 220 - age$$

There is no agreed-on best formula, and numerous scientists have tried to work out better mathematical regressions. All have a significant variation, but in reality, any will work as a starting point for your training. However, if possible, you should use the following method to better individualize your training.

**Measured Method:**

This method will give you a far more accurate result than the calculated method. Ideally, you should wear a heart rate monitor during the test, but if you can't get your hands on one, you can still use this technique and manually measure your pulse.

Perform the test on a home trainer or on a constant-grade road— either a level road or a consistent, mellow uphill. Eat 2 to 3 hours before the test, prepare your equipment, and be ready to suffer. After a 15- to 20-minute warm-up, follow these steps:

1. Start out at a moderate pace. You should be comfortable, but notably breathing. On a scale of 1 to 10, with 10 being maximal exertion, you should be at a 5 or 6.
2. Increase your speed by 1 mph every minute.
3. Shift when necessary, but avoid turning over a huge gear (you need leg speed to elevate your heart rate).
4. Suffer . . . and then suffer some more.
5. At your maximal effort, record your heart rate.
   - Heart rate monitor: Hit the record button or look at the file later.
   - Manual pulse: Immediately stop and measure your radial pulse for 15 seconds. Multiply this number by 4. (This will be slightly lower than your actual MHR because you had to stop to measure it.)
6. Repeat the test in 30 minutes. Follow the same steps.
7. The higher of the two numbers is your MHR.

## Power Meter Versus Heart Rate Monitor

| Power meter | Heart rate monitor |
|---|---|
| Instantaneous measurement | Time delay after effort |
| Actual measurement of performance | Measurement of physiologic response to effort |
| Quantifies training load by work | Quantifies training load by time in heart rate zones |
| Relatively expensive | Relatively inexpensive |

---

### Figure 3.4   Finding Your Maximal Power

You will need a power meter to perform this test. You should perform this test out on the open road, not on a home trainer. You'll be generating such a large amount of torque that many trainers can't support the effort. Now that's power!

Before you start the test, make sure you are comfortable with the functions of your power meter. Be able to recall the data so you can identify your power at maximal effort.

Find a straight section of road that is level or a mild to moderate uphill (preferably without many cars). Eat 2 to 3 hours before the test, prepare your equipment, and be ready to go hard! After an adequate 15- to 20-minute warm-up, follow these steps:

1. Do two intervals lasting 1 minute each.
2. Ride for 5 minutes at an easy pace.
3. Position yourself on a straight stretch of road. Start in the big chainring in the front, and slowly start to increase your speed. Keep your pedal cadence around 80 to 100 rpm.
4. Continue to shift to a smaller (harder) chainring in the rear until you increase your speed to a maximal sprint. It should take you about 30 seconds to reach your maximal speed.
5. Maintain your maximal sprint for at least 3 seconds.
6. Slowly recover. Ride easy for 5 to 10 minutes.
7. Repeat the test two more times.
8. The highest number is your maximal power.

# Sustained Performance

So far we've talked about the parameters that look at your maximal effort or your maximal potential. $\dot{V}O_2$max gives you the maximal amount of oxygen that you can consume as an athlete, and thus, the ceiling of your performance capability. Maximal heart rate gives a simple training measurement and approximation of the same. Maximal power shows exactly what the name implies—your maximal ability to apply torque to your cranks during your best and hardest effort. While maximal heart rate and maximal power both give you a practical measurement that you can use on the road, $\dot{V}O_2$max gives you a physiologic measurement in a sport laboratory.

Now, tuck all of that away but keep it available for reference. Many cyclists spend only a very small amount of time riding at their maximal effort. What they truly care about is just "riding faster" on the road. They want to put in a sustained effort and maintain a respectable velocity. That's where lactate threshold comes into play.

## Lactate Threshold Heart Rate

Let's talk about lactate threshold (LT). The burn. Natural ability and $\dot{V}O_2$max play a big role in your performance, but LT is much more interesting because it is highly trainable. A big part of any training program is taking your LT to the next level.

In chapter 2, we discussed aerobic (slow) and anaerobic (fast) metabolism. As mentioned, lactic acid is often used as an indicator for fast, anaerobic metabolism. Lactic acid was first discovered in sour milk by Carl Whilhelm in 1789. This is where it gets its name. Since that time, lactic acid has been a hot topic in sport physiology. As you work harder and harder—requiring more and more anaerobic metabolism (notably glycolysis)—you accumulate more and more lactic acid. This accumulation can be measured in a sport laboratory.

Remember, your body is always producing energy through both the aerobic and anaerobic systems. During normal life and easy intensity, the majority (but not all) of your energy comes from aerobic respiration. But even when you aren't killing yourself with a workout, glycolysis still contributes to the process, and as a result, some level of lactic acid is present. There is a balance, however. Your body constantly removes lactic acid and other waste products, preventing any accumulation of lactic acid.

Things change as your effort increases. As you raise your intensity, the rate of production of lactic acid also drastically increases. At some point, the system that removes lactic acid fails to keep up with production, and when that occurs, lactic acid begins accumulating in your blood. In the laboratory, the point at which lactic acid notably begins to accumulate is called lactate threshold, or simply LT. Other names for this include anaerobic threshold (AT) and onset of blood lactate accumulation. The historic term, *anaerobic threshold,* has fallen out of favor because we now know that the lactate threshold can occur even when there is ample oxygen delivery but not enough clearing of waste products.

Lactate is primarily a by-product of anaerobic or fast metabolism. As your muscles work harder and harder, they release an increasing number of protons, or hydrogen. You can think of hydrogen as acid. It creates "the burn." When another product of exercise, pyruvate, picks up these protons (hydrogen), it becomes lactate. So, contrary to popular belief, lactate is actually a marker, or by-product, of heavy muscle work, not the cause of muscle burn.

Textbooks often refer to the lactate measurement in the blood as lactic acid or lactic acidosis, but lactate is actually a short-term buffer, eating up excess hydrogen (taking acid out of the system). Thus, lactate actually slows acidosis. We still use the term *lactic acid* because it is commonly used in many training sources. When people talk about "lactic acid," what they are really referring to is the acid buildup from fast, anaerobic metabolism. The lactate level is really just an indirect marker that allows us to estimate the amount of anaerobic metabolism.

For years now, sport scientists have used this threshold point as a valuable physiological reference to compare one athlete with another and to compare changes in the fitness of a single athlete over time. The purpose of training, specifically interval training, is to improve your efficiency by *preferentially* using slow aerobic metabolism at ever higher workloads.

Even if the topic of LT seems foreign or new to you, you are undoubtedly aware of it from a practical standpoint. LT is the intensity level that causes you to feel the burn in your muscles. It's the point on your ride where you switch from talking about your night out on the town last night to focusing on getting your breaths in and out. The LT pace moves your ride from easy to hard.

## Confusing Terminology

**Lactate**—A good indirect marker of anaerobic metabolism.

**Lactic acid**—A term that is used interchangeably with *lactate* by many training sources. In fact, the body doesn't make true lactic acid, but the name has come to represent acid buildup from strenuous workouts.

**Lactate threshold**—The point when lactate production overwhelms lactate removal.

**OBLA**—An acronym for onset of blood lactate accumulation.

**Anaerobic threshold**—A term that is used interchangeably with *lactate threshold.*

LT represents the highest steady-state exercise intensity that you can maintain for an extended but fixed period of time, usually greater than 45 minutes but less than 2 hours. Your performance ability at LT is one of the best predictors of your endurance capability. In chapter 4, you'll learn how to use LT as a guide to your training intensity. I encourage cyclists to base their training on their LT rather than on their maximal heart rate, maximal power, or $\dot{V}O_2$max. Other coaches may have different preferences, and some use combinations of these values. There is a time and place for all the values laid out in this chapter, but when you're starting a new training program, your LT values can be used most effectively to set you up for success.

LT can be measured in the laboratory, on a trainer, or out on the road. In a sport laboratory, the LT test can be performed in conjunction with a $\dot{V}O_2$max test if so desired. While on a trainer, the athlete's power, heart rate, and potentially $\dot{V}O_2$ are all monitored. The rider begins a graded exercise test (as described in the $\dot{V}O_2$max section). Each stage of intensity lasts 2 to 6 minutes, allowing the rider to reach a steady-state heart rate, power, $\dot{V}O_2$, and lactate level. Blood samples are drawn (via finger prick) to determine the lactate concentration (millimoles per liter of blood, mmol/L). As the workload incrementally increases, so does the heart rate, power, and lactate concentration. At some point, the lactate concentration sharply increases. Other parameters, such as ventilatory effort, have been correlated with the sharp rise in lactate level. All parameters are recorded during the test and then graphed (figure 3.5).

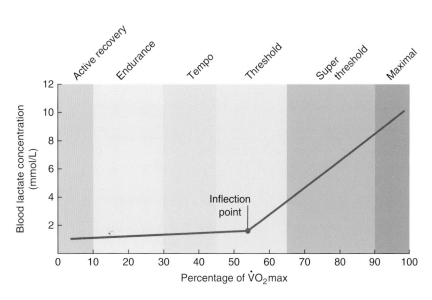

**Figure 3.5** Lactate threshold: During a graded exercise test, there is a point when the lactate concentration sharply increases. This is called the inflection point of lactate threshold.

## Lactate Threshold Power

By using a good training program, you'll see an increase in your LT levels. If the same athlete were to retest in the laboratory after a few months of training, there would be a shift in the lactate curve to the right (figure 3.6). This indicates that the athlete is producing the same amount of lactic acid while riding at a higher percentage of her $\dot{V}O_2$. This shift isn't notable only in the lab. When you achieve this shift, you'll also feel it on the road by tearing up the climb that used to kick your butt.

I mentioned my preference is that you base your training on your lactate threshold. All the intensity zones and workouts in this book are based on your personal values for LTHR (lactate threshold HR). Figure 3.7 shows how to find your LTHR. We'll be using these values in the later chapters.

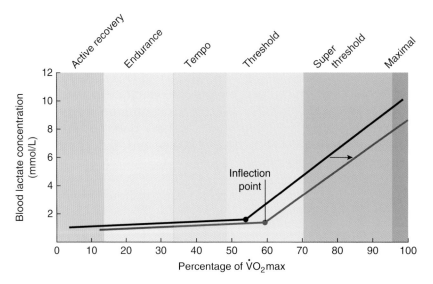

**Figure 3.6** Effect of training on lactate threshold: Training shifts the lactate concentration curve to the right. You are able to ride at a higher percentage of your maximum before the lactate threshold inflection point.

## Figure 3.7 Finding Your Lactate Threshold Heart Rate (LTHR) and Lactate Threshold Power

This test is a bit trickier than finding your maximal heart rate. You'll have to perform a constant effort for 30 minutes. The difficult part is finding the right speed. You want to go as hard as possible, at a constant intensity, for the entire duration. When you first do the test, you may have some variation in your effort. You'll start out too fast or too slow and then have to adjust. Don't worry if it takes you a couple of tries. You'll likely have to retest on a different day because the effort is so challenging. This test should feel difficult. Riding at your LT is no picnic. If you do it right, it hurts.

### Lactate Threshold Heart Rate

As with the maximal heart rate test, you can perform this test on a home trainer or on a constant-grade road—either a level road or a consistent, mellow uphill. Eat 2 to 3 hours before the test, prepare your equipment, and be ready to suffer. After an adequate 15-minute warm-up, follow these steps:

1. Start your stopwatch and begin your ride with a good cadence: 90 to 110 rpm.
2. Focus on breathing and settling into a mental zone. You want to be smooth and consistent.
3. Rate your discomfort every 5 minutes. This should remain fairly consistent throughout the test.
4. Record your heart rate over the last 20 minutes of your ride.
   - If you have a heart rate monitor, make sure you are either recording the event or documenting the heart rate at 5-minute intervals.
   - If you do not have a heart rate monitor, stop at 10, 20, and 30 minutes and measure your pulse. Immediately get back up to speed. Average these measurements to obtain your heart rate at lactate threshold (LTHR). Your numbers may be a little off compared to a heart rate monitor test because you have to stop intermittently.

### Lactate Threshold Power

Record your power over the last 20 minutes of your ride (this step is optional). Your average power over this interval will provide an estimate of your wattage at LT. Some cyclists use training zones based on their LT power.

To train efficiently and effectively, you must first know your baseline fitness. This allows your training to be graded and quantified. It also allows you to grade your progress. You'll get a fantastic feeling when you look back at your training log and see where you started and how far you've come. Different coaches and training methods rely on different parameters, but they all base their foundation on your maximal potential (performance ceiling) and your lactate threshold. Having a good understanding of these aspects will help you comprehend any training literature and work with any coach, regardless of the coach's specific techniques.

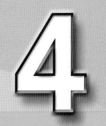

# Understanding Training Workload and Zones

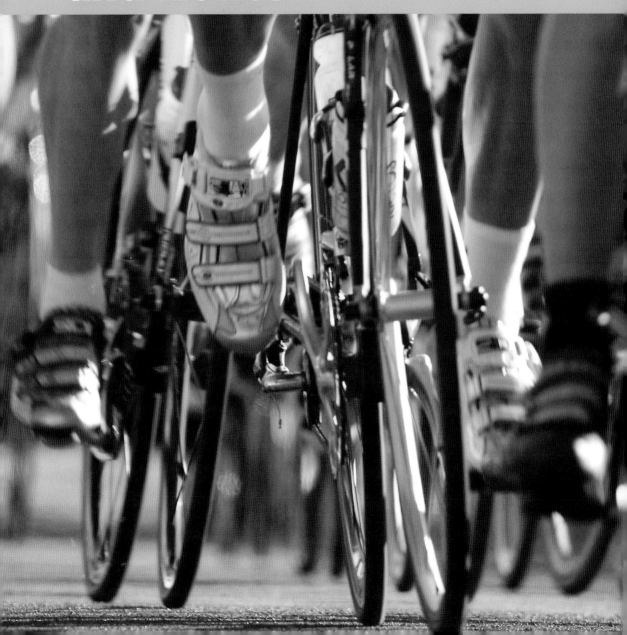

**It** is almost time to set up an actual training program and dive into the individual workouts provided in each of the specific training chapters of this book. But first, you need to have a clear understanding of how to quantify your training—specifically, how frequency, duration, and intensity relate to the overall stress that you place on your body.

Training is all about adaptation. You apply a load in hopes of getting a desired effect. The GAS (general adaptation syndrome) model shows that it is important to get the right amount of stress on the system. Remember the marshmallow from chapter 2? You want to apply just the right amount of heat to get the perfect marshmallow. The trick is to avoid both under- and overtraining. Every time you go out on your bike, you need to think about the alarm reaction, the adaptation from that alarm reaction, and the possibility of overtraining.

Ask yourself these questions:

Is this the right ride for how my body is feeling today?

Am I riding too often, not enough, or just the right amount?

How long should I ride today?

How difficult should I make my ride?

Do I have other big stressors outside of cycling that could contribute to the effort today?

All of these questions point to workload: frequency, duration, and intensity. This chapter breaks down each component individually and shows you how to quantify your training based on perception, heart rate, and power.

## Workload

Training workload, or training volume, is the stress you place on your body while working out. As a cyclist, you are always trying to apply just the right amount of stress. This is the fundamental difficulty of training. It's like the little girl who finds herself in the house of three bears: The stress you apply may be too much, too little, or just right.

Sport trainers are always in search of the "just right." But, it's no easy task. Athletes train their whole life trying to figure out how to cook the marshmallow without burning it.

Four variables make up the training workload: frequency, duration, volume, and intensity. During a training program, these variables can be mixed and matched in order to get the desired amount of stress on the system.

Here are some equations that represent workload and the components that contribute to your training effort:

$$\text{Workload} = \text{frequency} \times \text{duration} \times \text{intensity}$$

$$\text{Volume} = \text{duration} \times \text{frequency}$$

Simplified:

$$\text{Workload} = \text{volume} \times \text{intensity}$$

## Frequency

The more often you ride during a given cycle, the more stress you place on your body. When duration and intensity are kept constant, riding 6 out of 7 days in a microcycle is clearly a more difficult workload than riding 4 of 7 days. Because you can change each variable independently, you'll have the flexibility to fit various workloads into a hectic work schedule. You may only be able to ride 3 days a week, but by increasing the intensity and duration, you can complete a similar workload to someone who rides 5 days a week.

## Duration

A longer ride yields a larger training load. A 3-hour ride is more difficult than a 1-hour ride at the same intensity. Just as you have flexibility with the frequency of your rides, you can also adjust the duration of rides to arrive at your desired overall workload. Perhaps you have a busy schedule during the week, limiting the number of days you can ride, but on the days you do have free, you have the ability to do a longer ride. By increasing the duration of your rides, you can keep up the workload for the week. This technique has limitations, so don't go overboard. Deconditioning doesn't allow you to cram a week's worth of training into one Saturday. A break of 6 days will surely cause you to lose some fitness. But, you can be flexible within reason.

## Volume

Volume quantifies the frequency and duration of your rides. It answers this question: How much do you ride? Coaches and athletes use this number to track time on the bike. Some athletes know that they need a certain volume (e.g., 20 hours on the bike) before they really start to feel comfortable with intense training periods. Keep in mind that quantifying frequency and duration as a single product does have limitations. For example, you could go out for a 1-hour ride 5 days a week (5 × 1) or do one behemoth ride that lasts 5 hours on Saturdays (1 × 5). Both training programs would give you the same volume, but they may not give you the same training adaptation.

## Intensity

Intensity refers to the difficulty of your effort. An easy spin while talking with friends is low intensity. Breaking away on a final climb is obviously high intensity. Every ride in your training program is assigned an intensity, and by varying the intensity of your rides from easy to difficult, you'll add heat to the training flame. Some people believe that they have to ride as hard as possible on every ride. This is a mistake in the grand scheme of a training program. Intensity is just one piece of the overall training puzzle. Combining different frequencies and durations with a range of intensities will ultimately give you the best result.

Because it is easy to monitor and control the number of times you ride and the duration of your rides, intensity clearly becomes the trickiest of the three workload parameters to quantify. The remainder of the chapter shows you how to gauge your intensity and how to train using various *training zones*.

## Training Zones

Training zones are used to quantify and track intensity. Remember that workload is the product of volume (duration and frequency) and intensity. The volume component of your workload is easily tracked; all you need is a watch and a calendar. Intensity, however, is a whole different ball game. This is the toughest part of your training to get right.

As mentioned previously, every time you train you should have a goal for the workout. To reach that goal, you'll need to be aware of how hard you're riding (i.e., your intensity).

The purpose of a good training program is to work different aspects of your physiology. You'll be training your aerobic and anaerobic systems, your strength, and your mental fortitude. Some workouts may be for base training, building up the vascular machinery that will allow you to go hard later on. Other workouts may focus on training your maximal speed, allowing you to blow past a friend as you race for a city limit sign.

Each training zone represents a different level of effort, ranging from easy to hard. An overwhelming amount of information is available on training zones. Different coaches and books use different nomenclature, and this can make it confusing. This book is designed to give you a solid foundation in the world of training; the goal is to simplify things so that you'll have a good understanding that's adaptable to whatever terminology you encounter along the way.

Let's break intensity down into its simplest components. At the most basic level, you have to ask yourself a simple question before you head out on a training ride: "Is this workout easy or hard?" Is your bike rolling down the street with little effort, or are you about ready to blow a gasket?

Easy or hard. It's that simple. To focus on particular components of your physiology and to keep your workouts interesting, I further divide "easy" and "hard" into three different levels of workout intensity (figure 4.1). That gives you a total of six separate training zones (table 4.1).

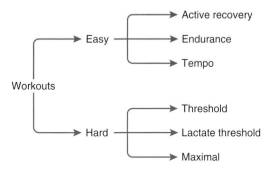

**Figure 4.1**  Easy versus hard workouts.

### Table 4.1   Training Zone Intensities

| Zone | Name |
| --- | --- |
| **Easy** | 1. Active recovery |
| | 2. Endurance |
| | 3. Tempo |
| **Hard** | 4. Lactate threshold |
| | 5. Super threshold |
| | 6. Maximal |

## Zone 1: Active Recovery

This is the easiest zone. It is intended to help you recover from difficult training rides. For example, you may train in this zone if you feel thrashed because you did multiple, high-end intervals the day before. An easy spin—while outside breathing the fresh air—can help you loosen and relieve tired muscles. The focus is to help your legs rejuvenate, and even though the training in this zone is easy, it's an important part of your overall training program.

## Zone 2: Endurance

Functionally, endurance work encompasses everything below your LT. The primary difference between recovery and endurance is the duration. On endurance rides, you will generally go longer and farther than a simple recovery ride. In the endurance zone, you should focus on laying the groundwork of your physiology so that you have a strong platform for your future training. All the blood vessels, capillaries, cells, and mitochondria need to be present before, as they say in the movie *This is Spinal Tap,* you "put it up to 11." Like any structure, your body is only as strong as its foundation, and that's what this training zone is all about. Early in the season, you'll spend a lot of time in this zone, but throughout the entire program, you should continually revisit your base conditioning.

## Zone 3: Tempo

A ride in the tempo zone is very much like an endurance ride, but with slightly more serious speed. You may stop to smell the roses on an endurance ride, but on a tempo ride, you need to be a little more focused and disciplined. This ride mimics a long effort, but it is done at an easier pace than when you're in a race or trying to obtain a personal goal performance. Focus on a rhythmic pattern, ticking away at the pedals and eating through the miles as you build up a solid physiologic foundation.

## Zone 4: Lactate Threshold

In this zone, you really hone in on trying to increase your LT. This is all about training your body to tolerate higher and higher intensities for longer periods of time. The less lactic acid you produce, the better you'll go on the road. You want your threshold percentage to be as high as possible. The purpose of this zone is to make your body efficient at using the available energy supply and enhancing the removal of cellular waste from exercise. It is a difficult training zone because it involves a hard effort that often lasts for an extended period of time. But once you start completing training cycles in this zone, you'll note the increased performance on the road. Fitness is a good feeling!

## Zone 5: Super Threshold

This is pure suffering. You will be counting the seconds (that seem like minutes) when doing intervals in zone 5. This intensity has you working above your LT. Your body is making the products of anaerobic metabolism faster than they can be cleared. You'll feel the burn building up right away. Zone 5 trains your maximal capacity and helps lift your $\dot{V}O_2$max. This intensity hurts, but the good news is that zone 5 intervals aren't nearly as long as zone 4; therefore, you can keep your mind focused on finishing the interval.

## Zone 6: Maximal

This is maximal effort. You'll be working in zone 6 when you sprint for the line or a hilltop finish. By definition, this intensity can only be maintained for short bursts. This is top-end output. Zone 6 training not only helps increase your performance ceiling, but it also helps you become "comfortable" at your high end. That might seem impossible, but you want to ensure that you don't go all spastic or lose form when you are sprinting for the line. Neuro-coordination goes out the window when you become very fatigued, and training in zone 5 and zone 6 will improve your ability to continue pedaling efficiently right when you need it most.

# Measurements of Intensity

The next obvious question is, How do you know which zone you are in while on a training ride? Well, the best way to quantify your intensity is to base it on your personal fitness. In the previous chapter, you learned how to determine your maximal effort and your lactate threshold. These are the concepts you will use to quantify your intensity.

## Rating of Perceived Exertion (RPE)

Many technological devices can be used to help guide your training. Heart rate monitors, power meters, and laboratory tests can all quantify your intensity. However, the first method to consider is the rating of perceived exertion. The RPE is an invaluable tool that is used by all levels of cyclists, from new athletes to professionals. As an added bonus, no equipment is needed! The RPE also happens to be one of the best measurements of your intensity level.

Introduced by Gunnar Borg, the RPE is a number scale that enables you to rate how "hard" you feel you are riding. Because of the name of the creator, the initial number rating system was sometimes referred to as the Borg index of perceived exertion. RPE is based on perception, not on an external number or data point. The rating is determined solely at the discretion of the rider. The perception of difficulty allows the rider to train in the specific training intensity zones described in the previous section.

Various RPE scales exist (with varying number designations), but a simple 1 to 10 intensity scale can be used very effectively. A rating of 1 is the lowest intensity—this represents a leisurely ride, chatting with a friend and just spinning. A rating of 10 is the other extreme, representing an eye-popping effort that puts you on the verge of a complete meltdown, vomiting and all.

Initially, using RPE is time and effort intensive because you have to teach yourself to distinguish between different levels of exertion based only on your perception. The key is consistency in the scale. Try to keep a 7 always a 7. Don't let other training devices such as a power meter or heart rate monitor sway you. If you think that your effort is a 7, then don't change that just because the heart rate monitor is putting you in a different training zone. The key attribute of the RPE is that it is a true rating of effort—of how you feel. Maybe you didn't get enough sleep, you have a huge work project, or you had a fight with your girlfriend or boyfriend. This all changes your effort and performance. An electronic device doesn't take into account the outside aspects of your life. RPE does.

| RPE scale | Sample feelings |
|-----------|-----------------|
| 1 | Recovery, merely stretching the legs |
| 2 | Spinning, lost in good conversation |
| 3 | Endurance training |
| 4 | Long ride, but a good workout |
| 5 | Requires focus, increased breathing rate |
| 6 | Heavy breathing, conversations end |
| 7 | Road race approaching a climb |
| 8 | Wondering how long you can last |
| 9 | Feel like quitting, dying, or winning |
| 10 | Eye-popping effort, nothing else matters |

Each RPE number will correspond to one of the training intensity zones (table 4.2).

Table 4.2    Training Zones and RPE

| Zone | Name | RPE |
|------|------|-----|
| Easy | 1. Active recovery | 1 |
|      | 2. Endurance | 2-3 |
|      | 3. Tempo | 4-5 |
| Hard | 4. Lactate threshold | 6-7 |
|      | 5. Super threshold | 8-9 |
|      | 6. Maximal | 10 |

## Lactate Threshold Heart Rate (LTHR)

Lactate threshold is another means for rating or quantifying your training intensity. As mentioned, at the most basic level, training would have two intensities: below LT (easy) and above LT (hard). LT draws the line in the sand. It represents a clear delineation in your workouts, and the better your LT, the longer you can "go hard."

Whatever your performance goal, the better your LT, the better your results. Training is all about being faster at a lower heart rate. It is about generating more power while putting out the least amount of effort. Being able to ride faster at or below your LT directly translates to improved performance on the bike. Your training goal should be to raise the bar. Get your LT as high as possible so you can go faster for longer without feeling the burn.

In the previous chapter, you learned how to find your personal LTHR and LT power. Each training zone can be defined as a percentage of your lactate threshold numbers (table 4.3).

Table 4.3   Training Zones and Percentage of LTHR

| Zone | Name | RPE | % of LTHR |
|---|---|---|---|
| Easy | 1. Active recovery | 1 | <80 |
| | 2. Endurance | 2-3 | 80-90 |
| | 3. Tempo | 4-5 | 90-97 |
| Hard | 4. Lactate threshold | 6-7 | 97-103 |
| | 5. Super threshold | 8-9 | 103-110 |
| | 6. Maximal | 10 | >110 |

## Lactate Threshold Power

$$Power = work \times time$$

Power meters are a tremendous training tool. Most professional cyclists have realized the benefit of including these devices in their training tool chest. If you use a power meter and you have performed the LT power test, you can use table 4.4 to base your training on a percentage of LT power.

Table 4.4   Training Zones and Percent of LT Power

| Zone | Name | RPE | % of LTHR | % of LT power |
|---|---|---|---|---|
| Easy | 1. Active recovery | 1 | <80 | <50 |
| | 2. Endurance | 2-3 | 80-90 | 50-75 |
| | 3. Tempo | 4-5 | 90-97 | 75-100 |
| Hard | 4. Lactate threshold | 6-7 | 97-103 | 100 |
| | 5. Super threshold | 8-9 | 103-110 | 100-150 |
| | 6. Maximal | 10 | >110 | >150 |

## Maximal Heart Rate

Using maximal heart rate as the reference for training zones is a common practice among coaches (table 4.5). The benefit is the ease of calculation. Remember, you can also use the following equation:

$$MHR = 220 - age$$

**Table 4.5  Training Zones and Percent of MHR**

| Zone | Name | RPE | % of LTHR | % of LT power | % of MHR |
|------|------|-----|-----------|---------------|----------|
| Easy | 1. Active recovery | 1 | <80 | <50 | <60 |
|      | 2. Endurance | 2-3 | 80-90 | 50-75 | 60-72 |
|      | 3. Tempo | 4-5 | 90-97 | 75-99 | 72-79 |
| Hard | 4. Lactate threshold | 6-7 | 97-103 | 100 | 80-90 |
|      | 5. Super threshold | 8-9 | 103-109 | 100-150 | 91-97 |
|      | 6. Maximal | 10 | >110 | >150 | >98-100 |

Figure 4.2 shows a quick and easy reference that enables you to get a quick start on your training before you are able to find any of your personal zones. It bases the training zones on your maximal heart rate, which in turn is based on your age.

| Exercise zones | | | | | | | | | |
|---|---|---|---|---|---|---|---|---|---|
| **Age** | | | | | | | | | |
| 20 | 25 | 30 | 35 | 40 | 45 | 50 | 55 | 65 | 70 |
| 200 | 195 | 190 | 185 | 180 | 175 | 170 | 165 | 155 | 150 |

**100%**

**Maximal**

| 194 | 189 | 184 | 179 | 175 | 170 | 165 | 160 | 150 | 146 |

**97%**

**Super threshold**

| 182 | 177 | 173 | 168 | 164 | 159 | 155 | 150 | 141 | 137 |

**91%**

**Lactate threshold**

| 158 | 154 | 150 | 146 | 142 | 138 | 134 | 130 | 122 | 119 |

**79%**

**Tempo**

| 144 | 140 | 137 | 133 | 130 | 126 | 122 | 119 | 112 | 108 |

**72%**

**Endurance**

| 120 | 117 | 114 | 111 | 108 | 105 | 102 | 99 | 93 | 90 |

**60%**

**Active recovery**

| 100 | 98 | 95 | 93 | 90 | 88 | 85 | 83 | 78 | 75 |

**50%**

Beats per minute

**Figure 4.2**  Maximal heart rate zones.

If you have the time and equipment, you should use RPE, percentage of LTHR, or percentage of LT power as the reference for training zones. All of these measures will be more accurate and efficient at training the various physiologic aspects intended by each intensity zone.

## Your Personal Training Zones

In the previous sections, you've seen how you can quantify your training intensity. To summarize, you should find your personal LTHR, LT power, and maximal heart rate. Plug these numbers into the charts in appendix A so that you can track your values over time.

Remember, as your training progresses, many of these numbers will change. As you become more fit, your heart rate at your lactate threshold will go up. This is exactly what you want. You can tolerate a higher and higher workload with less burn (inhibitory products of exercise). Your threshold heart rate and LT power will both go up with your fitness. Every few months, you may need to recalculate your actual numbers. Although the heart rate percentages remain the same for each zone, the actual numbers will change because you can tolerate more effort.

It is interesting to track the movement of your threshold heart rate as a percentage of your maximal heart rate. Divide your LT heart rate by your maximal heart rate and multiply by 100.

$$\text{Threshold percentage} = \text{LTHR} \div \text{MHR} \times 100$$

Over time, you can watch the gap between your LTHR and your maximal HR come down. You can do more work while making less and less inhibitory by-products. Performance goes up; burn goes down. For example, if your MHR is 180 and your initial LTHR is 150, then your LT is 83 percent of your max. If you train efficiently and effectively over the next few months, you may find that your new LTHR is 155 and your MHR is unchanged. In this case, you can clearly see the gains. You can now sustain an effort at 86 percent of your MHR.

You now have all the tools to start working on your personal training program. For effective training, you need to get the right workload. Now that you understand the concepts of frequency, duration, volume, and intensity, you can start the ongoing task of figuring out the perfect amount of training to meet your goals. Remember that every ride is part of the bigger picture of your training, and always keep in mind that the goal is to become a fitter, faster, and all-around better cyclist.

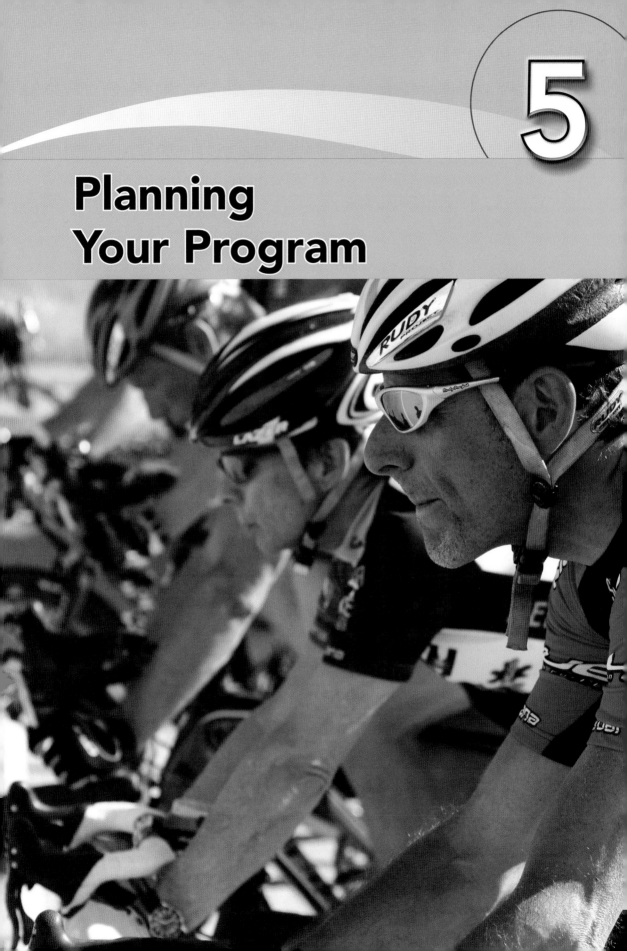

# 5

# Planning
# Your Program

**In** building a program, you need to bring all that we've discussed to the planning table. The RACE philosophy, adaptation, progression, and specificity all come into play when you are formulating a training plan. The entire training calendar revolves around these basic ideas. Based on the GAS (general adaptation syndrome) model, your program sets out a schedule of stress followed by rest. Your system is repeatedly "alarmed," and as a result, it adapts. Over time, the stressors are increased because your body is better prepared and adapted to the growing workload. This is exactly what you're hoping for—progression over time.

You'll spend the largest amount of your training time on the bike, focusing on specific cycling training. You'll also have periodic phases of crossover into other disciplines such as weightlifting, yoga, or running. These will help to improve and maintain your core muscles, your inherent strength, and your fitness. Rest, accountability, consistency, and efficiency hold the training system together and maintain the foundation that allows your fitness to soar.

You undoubtedly have questions running through your brain. How do you actually plan out a training program? How do you know when to apply the stress, how to determine if you're getting the desired response, and whether you are spending adequate time on specific cycling training? How do you know how much or how little to do?

The answers to these questions can be a little bit tricky. All athletes struggle with knowing how to reach their peak performance. No matter how long you train or how much information you inundate yourself with, there is always some uncertainty. You must simply do your best to design a well-thought-out, flexible plan. Each season will build on the last; you'll take everything you've learned and apply it to the new training year. The first year will likely be the most difficult, but with each added bit of experience, you'll start to feel more and more comfortable figuring out the best way for you to train.

The following sections describe how to use the information from the previous chapters to structure your step-by-step approach to ever more focused and demanding training. Again, the key to success is efficient training, and to make the most of your time, you need to be systematic and methodical in your training. Let's start by looking at periodization.

## Periodization

Periodization is a fairly simple concept. It involves building your training slowly and progressively, continually improving your fitness until you reach your ultimate goal. Tudor Bompa is known as the father of periodization, and his use of this training technique brought great success to the Eastern Bloc athletes for over three decades. Periodization uses a step-by-step approach, stacking one training phase or cycle on top of the other until you peak for your best performance (figure 5.1).

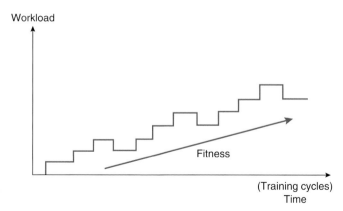

Workload

Fitness

(Training cycles)
Time

**Figure 5.1** Each training cycle builds on the previous one. In this step-by-step process of stress followed by rest, you gradually increase your fitness and ultimately your performance.

The training program includes a recurrent pattern: stress overload, followed by recovery, resulting in better and better performance. Individual training days are grouped into weeks, and these in turn are grouped into months. Each training day and each training cycle has its own specific goal, and all of these are designed to help you meet the ultimate goal of your training. For example, one cycle might focus on endurance, another on lactate threshold, and still another on climbing speed. When combined together they bring you from general fitness to your peak performance for the hill climb event you've marked on your calendar.

You begin to develop your periodization program by creating an annual plan. Chapter 1 discussed the importance of long-, medium-, and short-term goals. These will guide your entire program. Remember you can have multiple goals or "events" during the year. The annual plan is broken into various components, each representing different time periods of training (figure 5.2). The macrocycle is the largest period, encompassing the entire

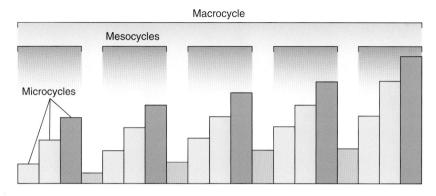

Macrocycle

Mesocycles

Microcycles

**Figure 5.2** Microcycles are the shortest training blocks. Multiple microcycles combine to make up a mesocycle. The mesocycle will have an overarching focus and goal, for example, improving anaerobic threshold. All the mesocycles are combined to make up the overall macrocycle.

plan. This is then broken into numerous mesocycles, each lasting 2 to 6 weeks. The training plan is further broken into microcycles, usually lasting about a week.

Some training plans and programs don't break their time periods into weeks or months. However, to keep things simple—especially with work, family, outside obligations, and weekends—you can use a calendar week as the fundamental microcycle.

The entire idea is to slowly improve, building on your previous workouts, all the while avoiding the possibility of overtraining. Periodization will keep your training focused. The various mesocycles will focus on different aspects of your riding, such as endurance, speed or as mentioned above, improving anaerobic threshold. The microcycles are still goal oriented, but they address the finer points of each mesocycle. Every training ride—and every micro- and mesocycle—should flow toward your ultimate goal. Each aspect of your plan should always follow the GAS model (alarm reaction, adaptation, exhaustion). Ideally, you continually move from days of stress to days of rest and adaptation. If you do it perfectly, you can avoid exhaustion and overtraining. Each day and cycle builds on your previous work. Over time, your body adapts to the entire training process, and you become stronger and faster—a riding machine!

When building a periodization program, you should work backward from your primary goal. Start with mesocycles, then fill in the microcycles, and finally work out individual training days. Remember, nothing is set in stone. As you train, your body will adapt, and this doesn't always occur according to a predetermined calendar. You need to listen to your body and adjust your training plan.

## Program Components

Your annual training plan will include three components, or general training periods: (1) Initial base phase, (2) Specific training phase, and (3) Transition. The microcycles build into mesocycles, which work toward each specific goal. The initial phase lasts 6 to 12 weeks, followed by a building or specific training phase lasting 2–6 weeks. During the specific training phase you'll hone in on the skills needed to complete your goals. Once you've completed your goal event, you move into the transition period. This allows your body to completely take a break before moving on to a new base phase.

Understanding all this terminology might seem a bit overwhelming, but once you get into a training program, you'll start to see how all the nomenclature makes sense. Just to recap, you have an annual plan that is broken into macro-, meso-, and microcycles. These are used to help you form a base, then build for performance, and ultimately transition to a new training goal.

To form a good periodization program, you must keep a few key points in mind. The first is that you need to outline a good set of goals. Next, you must be flexible. There is no way to avoid unforeseen changes in your training. Just as your physiology does with training, you'll have to adapt and modify your program based on life situations that may arise.

Always think of your program as working from the big picture to the fine details. Your training is always sharpening the knife to an ever finer cutting edge. Your program moves from large, nonspecific, low-intensity effort to very intense, highly focused training. The periodization program moves you from the general to the specific, and it makes sense from a workload perspective. High-volume, low-intensity effort creates a certain workload. High-intensity and low-volume effort also creates a certain workload (figure 5.3). If you continually couple high volume with high intensity, you'll surely burn out your engine. The workload would be too great. As stated earlier, periodization guides you through the GAS model so that you have just the right amount of stress to get maximal adaptation.

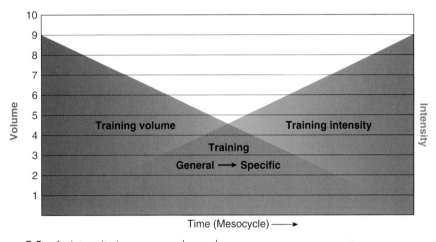

**Figure 5.3** As intensity increases, volume decreases.

## Fitness and Peak Performance

The purpose of your training program is to bring peak fitness at just the right time. The goal is to slowly progress, mixing fatigue and stress to bring about the best changes in your physiology. By using a periodization program, you can slowly increase your workload. Your body adapts accordingly and gradually increases fitness. You'll always be balancing your fitness level with fatigue. Your peak—the moment of your best performance—occurs when you can maximize your fitness and minimize your fatigue (figure 5.4). Only with a solid, methodical, and well-thought-out training program can you hope to have this occur at the time when you are approaching your goal.

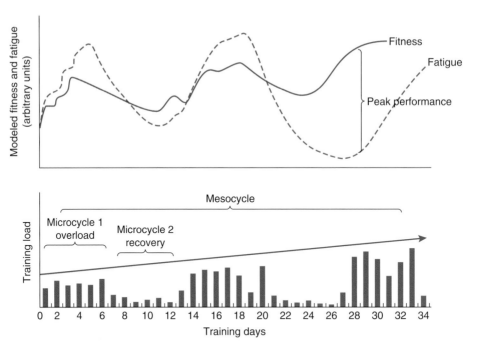

**Figure 5.4** Fitness, fatigue, adaptation, and peak performance. As you follow your training program, your body will become fatigued in response to the training load. As you recover, your physiology will gain a new level of fitness. This cycle will be repeated during your training program, gradually increasing your overall fitness. Peak performance, your goal event, occurs when your fitness level is at its apex and fatigue at its nadir.

## Training Diary

Track your progress, and over time your training will improve. By looking back at what you've done—where you've excelled and where you've faltered—you can make adjustments (some big and some fine) to your future training programs. A training diary is fundamental to a successful training routine. This applies to self-made training programs as well as prewritten programs like those found in this book.

The first step in creating the training diary is writing down your goals. You need to keep a good diary because no one can monitor yourself better than you. Only you can track the way you felt during a training ride. By combining subjective (what you feel) and objective (what is measured) data, you'll have a wealth of knowledge to guide your future training.

The training diary also enables you to document the components of the RACE philosophy. Rest, accountability, consistency, and efficiency are all monitored and evaluated in the training journal. Regardless of how technical

# Training Logs

by Dirk Friel, cofounder of TrainingPeaks.

A training log is a secret weapon for many cyclists, from Tour de France champions to recreational cyclists. A training log can grow with you as you develop as an athlete. The more you track, the more trends you may be able to spot. The real purpose of a log is to help you—and possibly your coach—replicate what worked and avoid what didn't go to plan. A log can help you predict the future and peak for your most important events.

Of course, training logs have changed over time, and what was once a hand-written journal has now evolved into new mediums. If you don't want to keep a hand-written journal, you have many web-based and mobile training logs to choose from. Migrating to the next generation of training logs provides a lot of benefits. It means you can track, analyze, and plan all aspects of your training from almost any computer or mobile phone in the world.

Not only can you track your training by manually entering your ride metrics, but you can also capture and record data in your log from a multitude of devices, such as power and heart rate monitors and GPS devices. Once the data are collected, you can use cutting-edge analytical tools to gain insight into where you could make marginal gains. It's not just about logging every workout—it's what you do with that data that produces results.

you want to make your diary, at a minimum you'll need to track basic progress (or lack thereof) toward your stated goal.

Any basic calendar can work as a training journal, but the best option is using a specific training log. You can purchase cycling-specific logs at your cycling shop or online, or you can make your own. There are also online training sites, such as Training Peaks, that help you organize your training (www.trainingpeaks.com). Dirk Friel, founder of Training Peaks, has made a career out of tracking training workload and progress.

Examples of simple and advanced logs are provided in appendix B. Sample logs are also available online at **www.HumanKinetics.com/products/all-products/Fitness-Cycling**. The simple log enables you to document all the ride parameters, such as time, distance, and intensity. The advanced log adds cadence, heart rate parameters, and power parameters. The spreadsheet allows easy data evaluation, graphing, and charting.

Here is a list of basic information that you should record in the simple and advanced logs:

**Simple:**

Date

Ride description

Distance

Time

Intensity

Emotional state (happy, sad, distracted, stressed)

Sleep

Fatigue level

Fitness level

**Advanced:**

All the information listed for the simple log

Average speed

Average cadence

Average power

Maximum heart rate

Average heart rate

Time in heart rate zones

Maximum power

Average power

Total work (in kilojoules/calories)

Your training log is a valuable tool for optimizing your performance. Again, your periodization program is about peaking for a goal. Your journal is a written description of your progress. After you reach the deadline for each personal goal, go back and look at what led to your success or failure. Try to find out where you went right and where you went wrong. Use what has worked for you in the past, and avoid the pitfalls that you've encountered previously. You'll enter each training year with a wealth of personalized information that will make your planning more efficient and effective.

# Getting Started

You've made it through all the basics of training. Now it is time to get out there on your bike and start training. This can all seem overwhelming if you're just getting started. But the workout chapters in this book are designed to make things easy on you.

Chapters 6 to 12 are arranged based on the various types of training. The workouts are provided as starting points. (Later, you can mix and match to make your own training programs.) The chapters cover various types of riding, such as sprinting, climbing, time trialing, and indoor training. Each chapter contains 8 to 10 workouts. For each workout, the description provided walks you through how to do that particular workout. A sample program is provided at the end of each chapter. You can use this as a guide to direct your overall training.

Start with the base-building workouts in chapter 6. This will give you the framework to do the other programs and hone your cycling skills and fitness. You don't have to do the workouts in the other chapters in any particular order. If you want to jump right in to climbing or time trialing, then just skip to the desired chapter. You should first do a couple of the programs just to see how your body settles into a training program.

After you have a good idea of your personal intensity zones and how to get through a particular program, it's time to step out on your own a bit. Take a calendar template and start to build your own program. Pick and choose workouts (from various chapters) that you like or that you think work well for you. Try to manage your workload so that you're not overcooking yourself. For the first program that you build, follow the color pattern (intensity zones) so that you're using a good mix of intensity.

Once you have that mastered, the training world is your playground. You can continue to use this book to pull out workouts to include in whatever training program fits your individuality, time constraints, and goals. Enjoy the workouts!

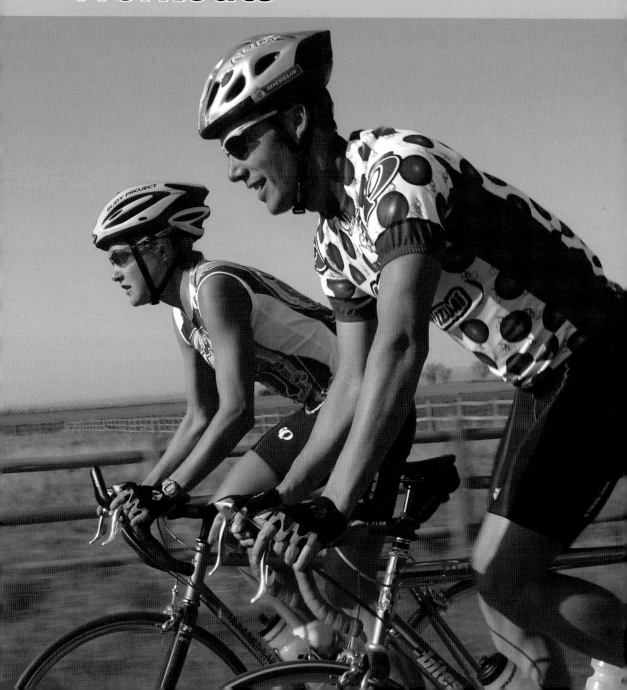

# Base-Building Workouts

# 6

# Tom Peterson's View

Tom Peterson is a member of Team Argos-Shimano Professional Cycling Team. He is a stage winner at the Tour of California and 4th overall at the Tour of Turkey. He also owns Peterson Bicycle Shop.

Every year starting in late November I bring cycling back to its roots and embrace the true essence of the sport. Even amid terrible weather I start to build up my miles and put in long casual rides solo or with friends. Stopping at coffee shops, trying new routes around the city and more than anything, enjoying the time I get to spend on my bike.

This is called base training. I love it, and I cherish most every moment of these rides. It's the one time of the year when I'm not doing intervals and killing myself. I can just enjoy riding around on my bike.

**This** is where it all begins. As the name implies, your foundation, or base, is at the very core of everything you'll be able to accomplish on your bike. All the fun stuff—riding fast, racing up a climb, completing a century—is rooted in the training from your base phase.

So what is *base*? Every endurance sport uses this or similar terminology to define the period of training when you're preparing your body to cope with increased workloads in future training. All the aspects of physiology discussed in chapter 2 come into play here. You are building up the energy supply, delivery, and output systems to do awesome work in the future. Good training is an accumulation of work over time. All of it matters in the future.

Whether you're just getting serious about cycling or you're a seasoned professional, your body will restructure during base training. The cardiovascular system lays down the framework for delivering a constant energy supply to your muscles so they can do work and turn the cranks on your bike. The better the underlying structure, the more stress it can handle in the future.

The Tour of Langkawi is a race held in Malaysia, and while going through Kuala Lumpur, riders get the opportunity to see the Petronas Towers. For a time these towers were the largest buildings in the world. They are 1,483 feet tall, and over 36,000 tons of steel was used in their construction. Because the bedrock was so deep under the towers, they have some of the world's deepest foundations. Within the steel and skeletal structure, miles of wiring, piping (for water, sewage, and sprinkler systems), and ducts (for air conditioning, heating, and venting) were routed throughout the entire structure. These elements make up the core of the building. During base training, you should think of the Petronas Towers. You are building all the required systems that will make your goal attainable. The Petronas Towers are awe inspiring, and your effort to reach your ultimate goal should be as well. Do the work now and reap the benefits in the future.

Base work is cumulative over the years. All the riding you've done in the past allows you to build your riding future. Just as each training block builds on the last for progression, each year of training progresses from the last. But that doesn't mean that after a few years you can skip this phase. True, a longtime pro has a bit shorter base phase than a new rider, but he still needs to build up his body after the off-season break. The base phase doesn't only apply to the beginning of the season either. If you have a long break because of injury, illness, or work, then you may have to revisit the base phase before you start heaping on the effort. Never try to go from zero to hero, especially because of impatience. This will only lead to a training disaster down the road.

Remember that one of the RACE training principles is consistency. The importance of sticking to the task and putting in the time at the beginning of your training season cannot be overemphasized. Consistency is what makes or breaks a training program, so take the base phase seriously. You are laying the foundation to build yourself up from a two-stroke go-cart engine into the big-block V8 that you want to be. Have faith in the fact that these early rides are making it all possible.

When you first start to do longer rides, you might finish a bit thrashed. Don't get discouraged by the way you feel on these early-season efforts. This is only the beginning. Remember, Sir Isaac Newton knew what he was talking about: An object at rest tends to stay at rest. Sounds similar to homeostasis. You are breaking the trend, moving in a new direction, and taking yourself out of your comfort zone. Take it day by day, and over the course of weeks and months, you'll realize that you are turning into a riding machine.

## Cycling Spotlight

Base training is a good time to start looking at your diet. Remember that you need to feed your engine high-quality fuel. In chapter 2, we discussed proper nutrition, and this is where you can start training yourself to eat properly. Look at your current weight and set a goal for where you'd like to be. Cycling long easy rides during the base phase will help you burn extra fat calories that may have accumulated before you started to get serious about your training. During the base phase, you are building up your body for future training and efforts. Always have plenty of food with you on your long rides. Long rides will help you figure out the best type of food to eat while on the bike (based on your particular palate). Always make sure you are starting your ride with the "tanks topped off." You have to think about the entire training cycle, not just the ride for today. Training is systematic; so is nutrition. Work on eating right, and your training will be optimized.

# COFFEE RIDE

Remember, during this base phase, it is all about consistency. Try to get out on the bike when you can, even if it is just 30 minutes on the trainer before work. And try to avoid "making up" training. Don't try to get all your training in on only Saturday or Sunday. That turns into just one big ride, and you lose the benefit of periodization and a training program.

| | |
|---|---|
| **Total Time** | 30 to 90 minutes |
| **Warm-Up** | Not necessary (easy ride) |
| **Terrain** | Flat to rolling |
| **Training Zone** | 1 |
| **Workout Time** | 30 to 90 minutes |
| **Cool-Down** | Not necessary |

This is a recovery or base-building ride that should be fun and social. Each training program is customized to the individual. Because of this, you'll spend the bulk of your time riding on your own. But not today! Meet some friends after a tough training week, or schedule this in the middle of a base-building block if you need some human interaction in order to keep from going off the deep end. Pick a cool place to stop for coffee and take a break. This can be anywhere during the course of the ride—beginning, middle, or end. It doesn't matter. Just hang out, get some miles in, and enjoy the company.

BASE-BUILDING

| | |
|---|---|
| **Total Time** | 45 to 80 minutes |
| **Warm-Up** | Easy spin for 10 minutes |
| **Terrain** | Depends on your city! |
| **Training Zone** | 2 or 3, with bursts of power |
| **Workout Time** | 30 to 60 minutes |
| **Cool-Down** | 5 to 10 minutes |

Today, you'll explore your city or town and the surrounding area. I used to have a great time riding my bike through Central and Riverside Parks when I was in medical school in New York City. Now I'm fortunate to have fantastic bike paths in Colorado. More and more communities are becoming cyclist friendly. Get out there and see what your home base has to offer. Even if there aren't specific bike paths, you should ride down smaller streets and explore your city. You'll get a great feel for the lay of the land and probably discover areas that you never thought of visiting. Play bike messenger for a day (like Kevin Bacon in the movie *Quicksilver*). Hone your bike-handling skills and stay alert. Watch for cars, obstacles, and hazards. DON'T GET HURT!

Work on your bicycle handling. Practice bunny hops, riding with no hands, and moving items in and out of your pockets. This is a no-stress ride, so have fun on the bike.

BASE-BUILDING

# HOLY ROLLER

Rotate your hand position during the ride. Place your hands on the handlebar tops, then on the hoods, and then on the drops. See how the ease of your riding changes, and, if you're watching your heart rate monitor, see if your heart rate changes based on position. Find your comfort zone. Some climbers like to sit for prolonged periods, while others like to be up out of the saddle and standing.

| | |
|---|---|
| **Total Time** | 50 to 80 minutes |
| **Warm-Up** | 10-minute spin |
| **Terrain** | Sustained climbs |
| **Training Zone** | 3 |
| **Workout Time** | 30 to 50 minutes |
| **Cool-Down** | 10 to 20 minutes |

The purpose of this workout is to give you saddle time on a sustained climb. Try to find a prolonged climb that you can settle into for 30 to 50 minutes. Keep your cadence up and the gearing easy. Try to control your heart rate so you don't go above zone 3 (tempo). Speed isn't important. Worry about your heart rate, form, and time in the saddle.

You may have to go up and come back down a couple of times. That's no problem—most of us don't live in the Rockies or Alps. If you have to ride down, keep pedaling at a similar cadence to your climb. Put power on the pedals as you descend. (As a bonus, you'll become more efficient at your descent technique.)

BASE-BUILDING

| Total Time | At least 2 hours |
|---|---|
| Warm-Up | Not necessary |
| Terrain | Variable. If you have to climb, go easy. |
| Training Zone | 2 |
| Workout Time | At least 2 hours |
| Cool-Down | Not necessary |

Don't forget sunscreen. Racers used to complain that the lotion prevented them from sweating properly. That's not the case any longer. Most riders lather up before long and sunny rides. Staying healthy and avoiding skin cancer far outweigh any imagined reduction in sweating capacity.

Today is the big day in your base training! This is where you go for a really, really long ride. The ride is difficult, not because of intensity, but because it is long. Your duration will go up as you become more fit. Don't overdo it at first. You want to avoid injuries, but you should definitely push your distance envelope. You're laying the groundwork for your future capacity.

Eat well and plenty during the days leading up to this ride. After each of your training rides, you need to eat promptly so that you are ready for the next day's training. If you get behind during the days leading up to the Big Boy, then you're going to have a difficult go of it. Bring plenty of food and sources of hydration on the ride, and make sure you have money so you can restock if necessary. (I hate to admit it, but I've been saved by a cold Coca-Cola on numerous occasions!)

You might prefer to find a loop rather than an out-and-back course for this ride. A loop makes the ride more entertaining and can intensify your commitment to making the distance. Consider riding to another city or a notable landmark, something that you can brag about when you're back at work. You'll feel gratified and proud when you park the bike after the Big Boy.

BASE-BUILDING

# GRANDMA

Always make sure that you have a well-stocked saddlebag full of the right items. This should include an extra tube, tire lever, patch kit, multitool, and two air cartridges. Also important is a stash of money. You never know when you might be starving and need a pick-me-up or when you might need to catch a bus home. I once had a three-flat ride in a thunderstorm. I managed to walk to a bus stop, only to be turned away by the bus driver because I had no cash! Fortunately, a compassionate soul and fellow rider let my dirty wet carcass into his car and gave me a lift home.

| | |
|---|---|
| **Total Time** | 1 to 2 hours |
| **Warm-Up** | Not necessary |
| **Terrain** | Flat |
| **Training Zone** | 1 or 2 |
| **Workout Time** | 1 to 2 hours |
| **Cool-Down** | Not necessary |

This is essentially a long recovery ride. Ride slow and easy. Don't watch the odometer because it will take you forever to get anywhere. This ride isn't about distance. It's about time on the bike. If other riders roll past and yell "Grandma," then you know you're doing it right. Focus on pedaling technique and the goals you've set for yourself. The ride might be slow, but it's building the foundation for future success.

BASE-BUILDING

| | |
|---|---|
| **Total Time** | Up to 1 hour 20 minutes |
| **Warm-Up** | 10-minute spin |
| **Terrain** | Flat, rolling, or hills (It's all good!) |
| **Training Zone** | 3 |
| **Workout Time** | Up to 1 hour |
| **Cool-Down** | 10 minutes |

This ride should be just below your lactate threshold. You want to try to hold a steady tempo throughout the ride. Try to keep your heart rate controlled. During races, team directors will tell their riders to go to the front and "ride at tempo." They want their racers to hold a good pace without paying too much from the energy bank account. Remember, if you are below your LT, you should be using a large portion of your energy from fat. Tempo riding allows you to maintain a respectable pace with the capacity to pick it up a notch if the terrain or race requires it.

Train yourself to take a drink at least every 15 minutes. If you have trouble remembering, set a timer with an alarm. You want to form a good habit of regularly reaching down for your bottle, even before you feel thirsty. Obviously, hydration requirements change based on the conditions, but a general rule is to shoot for drinking one bottle per hour.

# SLOW RIDER

Before this ride, you should complete this homework assignment: Go online and watch some videos of professional cyclists while they climb. Notice their smooth leg circles as they pedal. Their heel remains low as they apply pressure through their entire cadence. Try to emulate the professionals' form while you do these slow-motion intervals.

| | |
|---|---|
| **Total Time** | 1 to 2 hours |
| **Warm-Up** | Not necessary |
| **Terrain** | Flat |
| **Training Zone** | 2 |
| **Workout Time** | 50 minutes to 2 hours |
| **Cool-Down** | Finish the ride with an easy spin for at least 10 minutes. |

You're going to be doing intervals during this ride, but they are not based on intensity. They're all about pedaling technique. Do 10-minute intervals using a super-slow cadence. If you normally ride using a cadence of 85 to 100 rpm, these intervals are done in the range of 55 to 65 rpm. Focus on pedaling throughout the entire revolution. See chapter 14 for proper pedaling technique and force application. Make sure you have some base miles under the tires before trying the Slow Rider. Because of the increased torque, this workout puts more strain on ligaments and tendons.

| | |
|---|---|
| **Total Time** | 1 to 2 hours |
| **Warm-Up** | As dictated by the group |
| **Terrain** | Flat |
| **Training Zone** | 3 or 4 |
| **Workout Time** | 1 to 3 hours |
| **Cool-Down** | As dictated by the group |

This is group training, and you're going along for the ride! First, I should explain the odd name of this workout. When I used to be a racer myself (long, long ago), we would always ride out to Canalow every Wednesday. This was a group ride where riders could test themselves against everyone else. To this day, whenever I think of a group ride, I think of Canalow. After you find your own Canalow, I'm sure you'll change the name.

Find a good group ride in your area. Check at local bike shops to see when and where people are meeting. Ideally, this ride should be 1 to 2 hours. Try to avoid short group rides, because they often turn into a speedfest, which is not what you're looking for here. It is OK if the riders turn up the pace; just don't get carried away in a criterium or sprint event.

Don't "half-wheel" anybody on a group ride. Half wheeling is when you continually inch your bike ahead of the rider who is next to you. This results in a faster and faster pace over time as your partner tries to keep his wheel in line with yours. Good etiquette dictates that you must keep your front wheel even with your partner's front wheel when riding side by side.

BASE-BUILDING

Gearing helps your efficiency. Just like with a car engine, changing gears lets you perform optimally. As a general rule, when riding harder, you should match the burn in your legs to the burn in your lungs. Increasing your cadence will increase the burn in your chest but decrease the burn in your legs. Vice versa, decreasing your cadence and using more torque will decrease the burn in your lungs but increase the pain in your legs.

| | |
|---|---|
| **Total Time** | 1 to 2 hours |
| **Warm-Up** | Not necessary |
| **Terrain** | Flat |
| **Training Zone** | 2 or 3 |
| **Workout Time** | 50 minutes to 2 hours |
| **Cool-Down** | 10 minutes at an easy, normal cadence |

High cadence is all the rage . . . or in this case, *rave*. Train with a good cadence and you'll become more efficient and adept at keeping your pedaling rpm up when you start to go hard. Old-time professionals rode with a slow cadence, but for the past 10 years, most elite climbers and racers find the higher cadence more efficient. Just look at any stage in the Tour de France and pay attention to the front group riding up a Hors catègorie climb.

This ride is the opposite of Slow Rider. During this ride, you should do 10-minute intervals of a quick cadence. If you normally ride using a cadence of 85 to 100 rpm, your intervals should be done in the range of 115 to 120 rpm. Focus on technique and being smooth. With faster cadences, riders have a tendency to bounce a bit in the saddle. Try to relax your leg muscles, letting them spin through their revolutions. Smooth and calm. That's your goal.

| | |
|---|---|
| **Total Time** | 1 to 2 hours |
| **Warm-Up** | Not necessary |
| **Terrain** | Flat |
| **Training Zone** | 2 |
| **Workout Time** | 1 to 2 hours |
| **Cool-Down** | Not necessary |

This ride is nothing fancy, but it serves a very important purpose. You will use the Long Recovery ride a bit later in your training. During the weeks with hard efforts, you'll need to take a break and recover. This ride will help you maintain some good endurance while at the same time letting the muscles recover. There is no structure to this ride other than keeping it really easy. You can talk with friends, zone out to some music, or do anything else that helps provide a bit of rest for your weary body.

Use chamois cream when doing longer rides. This might take a little getting used to, but in the long run, it will help you avoid saddle sores. Apply the cream liberally to your crotch when putting on your cycling shorts. Remember to shower as soon as possible after your ride. Always clean your shorts before rides, and ideally, let them dry out of the sun in the open air.

## Sample Base Program

| Week | Mon | Tues | Wed | Thurs | Fri | Sat | Sun |
|------|-----|------|-----|-------|-----|-----|-----|
| 1 | Off or gym | Long Recovery Pg. 69 | Long Recovery Pg. 69 | Off or gym | City Cruise Pg. 61 | Coffee Ride Pg. 60 | Rave Pg. 68 |
| 2 | Off or gym | Long Recovery Pg. 69 | Tempo Pg. 65 | Off or gym | Slow Rider Pg. 66 | Holy Roller Pg. 62 | Grandma Pg. 64 |
| 3 | Off or gym | Long Recovery Pg. 69 | Tempo Pg. 65 | Off or gym | Rave Pg. 68 | Tempo Pg. 65 | Big Boy Pg. 63 |
| 4 | Off or gym | Holy Roller Pg. 62 | Long Recovery Pg. 69 | Off or gym | Slow Rider Pg. 66 | Canalow Pg. 67 | Grandma Pg. 64 |
| 5 | Off or gym | Tempo Pg. 65 | Tempo Pg. 65 | Off or gym | Rave Pg. 68 | Grandma Pg. 64 | Big Boy Pg. 63 |
| 6 | Off or gym | Coffee Ride Pg. 60 | Holy Roller Pg. 62 | Off or gym | Long Recovery Pg. 69 | Canalow Pg. 67 | Big Boy Pg. 63 |

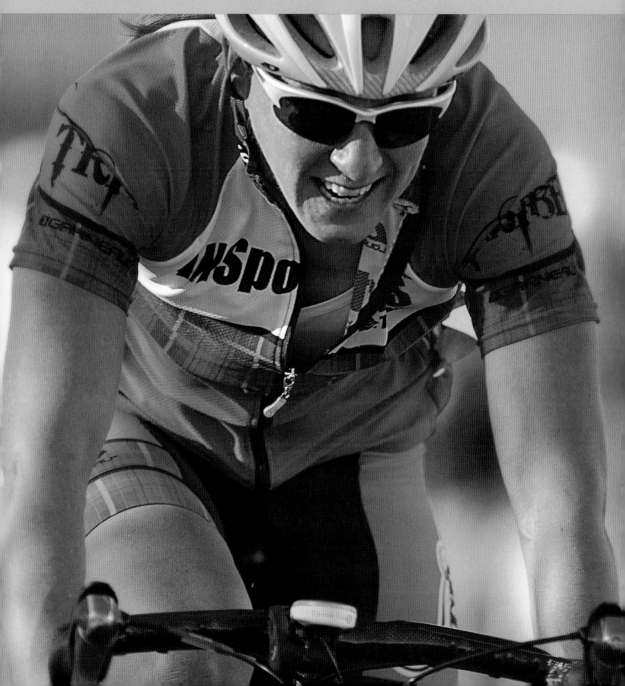

# Interval Workouts for Flat or Varied Terrain

# 7

# Taylor Phinney's View

Taylor Phinney is a member of the BMC Professional Cycling Team. He won stage 1 of the 2012 Giro d'Italia and was also an Olympian in 2012.

Some cyclists ride their bike just because they love it. They ride in a completely unstructured training environment, purely because riding a bike provides that beautiful escape that we all know and love. Riding for the love, as I like to call it, not only does the body good but also the mind.

This type of riding is necessary for even the most serious professionals. But if you wish to raise your game—if you wish to step up to that next level and become a race winner, or even just that guy who throttles everyone on the Saturday group ride—you must do interval training. Cyclists who ride for the love will soon reach a fitness plateau because of the lack of structured training. As much as I love just going out and riding my bike, I know from experience that on most of the days that I call training days, I am going to have to do intervals. The only way you can build on your current foundation is to train very specifically for what you are trying to achieve—which means doing intervals.

I'll give you an example. I have always considered myself a time trialist, but more of a short time trialist specializing in events between 15 and 20 minutes. In 2011, I won the 5-kilometer prologue at a World Tour stage race called the Eneco Tour. But at the 2011 World Championships in Copenhagen, when I competed in a 46-kilometer time trial against the best in the world, I couldn't match the pace and only managed 15th place.

The summer of 2012, I got called up to represent the United States at the London Olympics in both the road race and the time trial; the time trial would be my main focus, although it was at a distance of 44 kilometers, much longer than what I would normally be comfortable with. The day I heard of my selection, I sat down with my coaches, and we formulated a plan. The plan involved very specific intervals in an attempt to turn the world's 15th-place time trialist into a medal contender in the Olympic time trial. The intervals I completed over the following weeks leading up to the Games were hellish to say the least. It was blistering hot in Boulder that summer, and I would be out for 3 to 4 hours on my TT bike, working harder and more specific than I ever had before. The gains were massive and immediately noticeable week after week. I went to the Games more prepared than ever, and I just missed out on a medal, finishing in a respectable 4th place. The work I did that summer carried over into the 2012 World Championships in September, where I finished an even better 2nd place, missing that rainbow striped jersey by only 5 seconds (over a distance of 46 kilometers). Going from 15th to 2nd in one year is a big jump, but it was the result of my very specific interval training regimen that was crafted only months earlier.

**You're** going to love these workouts! OK, maybe you'll love them and hate them at the same time. These training days are difficult. They're a struggle to get through, and the goal is to make you suffer—sometimes a little, sometimes a lot. But that is why you'll love them. You'll get a real sense of achievement after you finish.

As mentioned, the base training in the previous chapter was designed to lay the foundation for all the workouts in later chapters. Now you'll be getting into the meat of your performance training. These workouts train the limits of your aerobic energy supply and the efficiency of your anaerobic system. Your goal here is to increase your lactate threshold—the higher your threshold, the better your performance.

Maybe you've seen the movie *This is Spinal Tap*. Referring to his awesome amp, Nigel says, "But this one goes to 11." Imagine how fast you would ride if your threshold was the same as your maximal heart rate. Turn it up to 11, full power, and go.

The reality is that you can't do that. Nobody can. You can sustain your maximal power output for only seconds at a time. Not even the greatest cyclists in the world are gifted with the ability to ride maximally for an extended period. But, your goals for training should focus on trying to bring your lactate threshold as high as possible. Your $\dot{V}O_2$max (maximal heart rate) is the limit. The closer you can move your LT to $\dot{V}O_2$max, the faster you'll go for a longer period of time.

The workouts in this chapter will help you raise your LT. Numerous kinds of "threshold" workouts are available. The range of workouts provided here will not only train your aerobic and anaerobic systems, but will also keep things spicy so you can keep your mind off the effort—off the pain.

These workouts hurt. Nothing comes for free, and if you want to increase your ability to sustain a fast pace, then you're going to have to work on suffering. Professional cyclists are all about suffering. That in itself makes them an odd lot. They are like sadistic monks, and that's why they get paid the big bucks. You don't need to go out there and kill yourself, but you will have to work hard and focus on completing the workout.

You should be proud of yourself when you complete these workouts. Completing a set of intervals is an accomplishment. You'll find a whole new appreciation for a chair or couch. As cyclists always say, "Why stand when you can sit? Why sit when you can lie down?" You'll be saying the same thing when you finish training your lactate threshold.

Regardless of your fitness goals, interval training is a necessary component of your workouts. This chapter isn't just for racers. Anyone who wants to ride faster, perform better, lose more weight, or just challenge herself needs to focus on interval training.

# Interval Basics

In concept, intervals are quite simple. They are workouts with alternating periods of effort and rest. Where things get tricky is in the details. How many intervals should you do? How much effort and rest? How often do you do interval training? These are the questions that continually plague athletes and coaches. This section describes some basics that will provide you with general rules to follow when setting up workouts. You can also refer to the sample program at the end of the chapter to see an example of how to incorporate intervals into your overall program.

Like all the workouts in this book, you can base your interval training on multiple intensity parameters. RPE, LTHR, LT power, and MHR can all be used to guide your training. The workouts identify the specific zone for training and allow you to choose the method of intensity measurement.

In general, the rest period is related to the work period and intensity. The shorter the interval, the harder the intensity. Because you'll be performing at such a high level, the shorter intervals require longer periods of rest. Longer intervals—those that involve training more in the aerobic zones (tempo)—require less rest because they don't involve the super intense effort that places you in so much debt.

The workouts in this chapter are set up based on intensity and one of two modes for measuring recovery:

1. A predetermined rest period
2. A reduction in HR to a percentage of LTHR or MHR

# Interval Shorthand

Many coaches use a shorthand when writing down interval workouts. Perhaps you've seen something similar to this: 1 × 3 × 10. How do you decipher these numbers? The first number is the length of the interval (minutes or seconds). The second is the recovery time (minutes or seconds), and the third is the number of intervals to be performed. Thus, 1 × 3 × 10 means a 1-minute effort, followed by a 3-minute rest. The workout requires 10 intervals. Note that the relationship of effort to rest is often referred to as a ratio. In this instance, the interval is a 3:1 rest-to-effort ratio.

Interval training is fundamental to any effective training program. The efforts are difficult, but they give you a lot of bang for your buck. You will suffer, but you'll be a much stronger and fitter cyclist because you put in the time doing intervals.

## Cycling Spotlight

Remember, the two fundamental training levels are easy and hard. Most of these workouts fall into the hard category. You will be giving efforts at or above your LT. Some workouts are designed to give you good recovery between efforts, and others purposefully commence a new effort before you feel ready. It's all part of developing your physiologic efficiency and raising your lactate threshold.

Each method has its advantages. The predetermined time method is easier to use. You don't have to worry about using a heart rate monitor or tracking your heart rate during recovery. You merely have to look at your cycling computer stopwatch. Intervals based on a percentage of your heart rate are beneficial because they base your interval on your physiologic response rather than an arbitrary amount of time. The downside is that this method is slightly more complex and requires a heart rate monitor.

For this book, the interval workouts are based on time. This will expose you to the various types of interval workouts without the complication of needing to make calculations of recovery based on a heart rate monitor. Any of the interval workouts can be adapted to allow the use of a measured recovery if you desire in the future.

Get used to being uncomfortable. These workouts are a challenge. Most people don't know what it feels like to give a 100 percent effort. Once you experience the uncomfortable feeling of pushing to the maximum, you'll be able to better understand your true capability. Most people can push themselves harder than they think. By stretching your effort out of the comfort zone, you'll see marked improvement and fitness gains.

(30 seconds × 90 seconds × 8)

| | |
|---|---|
| **Total Time** | About 50 minutes |
| **Warm-Up** | 15-minute spin |
| **Terrain** | Flat or rolling hills |
| **Training Zone** | 6 |
| **Workout Time** | 16 minutes (4 minutes at zone 6) |
| **Cool-Down** | 20 minutes |

Get ready and go! These are "full-gas" intervals. Make sure you perform a good warm-up. Before you push it into zone 6, ride a few minutes of your warm-up in zone 4 or 5.

You will give your best effort for 30 seconds, followed by 90 seconds of rest. Perform a total of 8 cycles of work–rest.

Keep a good cadence throughout the interval, and don't push an overly difficult gear. Do these intervals in your handlebar drops and work on keeping your upper body smooth. Earlier this week, I was watching the final kilometers of a stage of the Giro d'Italia from the team car. Based on the riders' form and upper-body movement, I could see who from the team was "going good" and who was "on the rivet." Christian Vande Velde's shoulders were so smooth and steady. He closed a gap to the leaders from 4 minutes to 1 minute in a matter of 5 kilometers . . . by himself!

These intervals have a 3:1 rest-to-effort ratio. You'll go as hard as possible for 30 seconds and then let your body recover before trying another effort. This is high-intensity training, so fasten your seat belt and gun the accelerator. Notice that you only have 4 minutes of "go time"; the remaining time is warm-up, effort recovery, and cool-down.

INTERVAL

76

(45 seconds × 5 minutes × 4)

| | |
|---|---|
| **Total Time** | About 45 to 50 minutes |
| **Warm-Up** | 15-minute spin |
| **Terrain** | Flat or rolling hills |
| **Training Zone** | 6 |
| **Workout Time** | 18 minutes (3 minutes at zone 6) |
| **Cool-Down** | 10 to 15 minutes |

| Effort | Rest |
|---|---|
| 45 seconds | 5 minutes |
| 45 seconds | 5 minutes |
| 45 seconds | 5 minutes |
| 45 seconds | Cool-down |

This is a simple 45-second interval followed by a long period of recovery. It doesn't seem like a lot of work, but you should focus on getting the absolute most out of your body on each interval. Consider this a 45-second race for everything that's important to you.

Keep your form throughout the interval. Don't switch positions once you start. You should be going so hard that you wish you'd get a flat tire so you could stop early.

With a 5-minute rest, you should be well recovered before you start your next interval. The total time of this workout is short, so it is a good choice if you're on a tight time budget during the week.

Get into a routine of fueling before your workouts. If you don't take care of yourself off the bike, then you won't get the most out of your time on the bike. Ideally, you should have a light bite to eat about 1 to 1 1/2 hours before the workout. Eat a bar, banana, or yogurt. You can experiment to find out what makes you feel and ride the best.

Be sure to have clean shoes! Pros love clean shoes. Enter any team bus before a race and you'll see all the riders cleaning their shoes with wipes. This may or may not make you go faster, but clean shoes will certainly give you more style points. When you look down at your feet spinning through the rotation of the crank, perhaps clean shoes will give you just a little extra boost. That's one of the secrets of the pros.

(15 seconds × 15 seconds × 8)

| | |
|---|---|
| **Total Time** | About 50 minutes to an hour |
| **Warm-Up** | 15-minute spin |
| **Terrain** | Flat or rolling hills |
| **Training Zone** | 6 |
| **Workout Time** | 12 to 17 minutes (7 minutes 30 seconds at zone 6) |
| **Cool-Down** | 20 minutes |

These are fast on, fast off intervals. You'll be rapidly switching between going ballistic and just spinning: 15 seconds full power, 15 seconds rest. After 8 cycles of effort and rest, you can take a break for as long as you need in order to feel recovered (likely between 5 and 10 minutes). Then you are back at it for one more go-around, completing the entire 8 intervals again.

As mentioned previously, the higher intensity intervals generally need longer rest periods (often 2:1 or 3:1 ratios). However, there are always exceptions. This workout is specifically designed to put you into a worse and worse state of fatigue as the intervals progress. You are training your body to adapt to the higher level of waste products that will be accumulating after each interval.

Feel free to stand or sit during the periods of effort, but try to mix it up to keep your body guessing. Remember, the body likes homeostasis; it likes to know what is coming next. Your job is to keep your physiologic systems guessing.

During the periods of rest, focus on exhaling in a controlled and regular manner. Many beginning athletes are too worried about getting the air into their lungs. On the contrary, your focus should be on controlled exhalation, breathing off all the excess carbon dioxide. The inhalation part will come automatically as you establish a controlled rhythm.

INTERVAL

(1 minute × variable × 8)

| | |
|---|---|
| **Total Time** | 50 minutes to 1 hour |
| **Warm-Up** | 15-minute spin |
| **Terrain** | Flat or rolling hills |
| **Training Zone** | 4 or 5 |
| **Workout Time** | 22 minutes (10 minutes in zone 5) |
| **Cool-Down** | 20 minutes |

| Effort | Rest |
|---|---|
| 1 minute | 30 seconds |
| 1 minute | 45 seconds |
| 1 minute | 1 minute |
| 1 minute | 1 minute, 15 seconds |
| 1 minute | Take a break for 5 to 10 minutes |

During Minutemen, the effort period remains unchanged for all the cycles of effort followed by rest. But, the rest period progressively lengthens. This is because you will likely recover faster after the first interval than you will after the fourth. With each successive round, you'll get a slightly longer period of rest. If you performed minute-long intervals with a heart rate monitor guiding your recovery, you would likely see a similar pattern of successively increased durations of rest to bring your heart rate down to the desired pre-effort level.

Why stand when you can sit? Why sit when you can lie down? High-performance riders are always worried about recovery. If you are doing high-energy intervals a couple of times a week, you need to focus on letting your legs recover. Remember, your adaptation occurs while you are at rest, not during the workout!

INTERVAL

# DOUBLE TIME

You can use mental tricks to help you make it through intervals. One trick is to switch your hand position every 30 seconds. This is a short-term mental goal that helps get you to the next step of the interval. For example, start on the drops of the handlebar, move to the hoods, then to the tops, and then back down to the drops for the finish. This will also make you more smooth in transition when changing positions.

(2 minutes × 2 minutes × 4)

| | |
|---|---|
| **Total Time** | About 1 hour |
| **Warm-Up** | 15-minute spin |
| **Terrain** | Flat or rolling hills |
| **Training Zone** | 4 or 5 |
| **Workout Time** | 14 minutes (8 minutes in zone 4 or 5) |
| **Cool-Down** | 20 minutes |

| Effort | Rest |
|---|---|
| 2 minutes | 2 minutes |
| 2 minutes | 2 minutes |
| 2 minutes | 2 minutes |
| 2 minutes | Cool-down |

Have you ever felt as if time was slowing down? Well, with Double Time intervals, you'll feel as if two minutes is forever! You'll have to perform the two-minute interval in the upper level of zone 4 or the lower level of zone 5. As with all the intervals, you should focus on your breathing, specifically exhalation. Try to distribute power throughout the entire pedal stroke.

After completing a cycle of these intervals, you'll gain a lot of confidence in your ability to put the hammer down when cresting the top of a hill, riding up to a finish line, or just plain sustaining power when pulling away from your friends.

(variable)

| | |
|---|---|
| **Total Time** | About 1 hour |
| **Warm-Up** | 15-minute spin |
| **Terrain** | Flat or rolling hills |
| **Training Zone** | 4 or 5 |
| **Workout Time** | 14 minutes (8 minutes 30 seconds in zone 4 or 5) |
| **Cool-Down** | 20 minutes |

| Effort | Rest |
|---|---|
| 30 seconds | 30 seconds |
| 45 seconds | 45 seconds |
| 1 minute | 1 minute |
| 2 minutes | 10-minute rest |

Workups are tough because you know that you will keep getting progressively longer and longer interval periods. You won't have quite enough time to recover from the last interval before you have to start the next period of effort. Stay focused and do your best, maintaining your full commitment throughout the entire effort. You'll do two complete cycles.

Think about how your fitness is improving. You're putting a big stress on your system. Work-ups definitely trigger an alarm reaction (you'll know it after you complete the first cycle when you feel like crying). But, as a result of this stress, your body will start making adaptations when you rest. You'll slowly be getting faster, stronger, and more fit because you're putting in the time. Nothing comes for free, and the cost of fitness is struggling through your interval program.

During the 10-minute rest, make sure that you are taking an easy spin on the bike. You'll recover faster if you let your legs spin easy rather than just stop completely. This is true after any hard effort. Focus on keeping your legs moving, even if you are exhausted. The motion will enhance energy delivery and waste removal from your legs.

INTERVAL

Always check your brakes, tire pressure, and other equipment before you ride. Even if you have a pro mechanic fixing your bike, you'll be the one who is trusting it to work properly. Checking the equipment takes 30 seconds, but it could save you while out on your ride.

(variable)

| | |
|---|---|
| **Total Time** | 45 minutes to 1 hour |
| **Warm-Up** | 15-minute spin |
| **Terrain** | Flat or rolling hills |
| **Training Zone** | 5 |
| **Workout Time** | 13 minutes (8.5 minutes in zone 4 or 5) |
| **Cool-Down** | 20 minutes |

| Effort | Rest |
|---|---|
| 2 minutes | 30 seconds |
| 1 minute | 45 seconds |
| 45 seconds | 1 minute |
| 30 seconds | 10-minute rest |

Workdowns require that you pace yourself. You have to start the first 2-minute interval using an effort level just under the level that you used during the Double Time workout. You have a reversed rest interval, so you can't spend all your energy in the first 2 minutes.

Workdowns are a bit less mentally challenging than Workups because each effort period is getting shorter and shorter. That gives you hope during your training session. Intervals are all about laying it on the table and giving it what you've got. Don't be demoralized if you are not going gangbusters during your last 30 seconds. The point is that your *effort* is maximal. You are training, not performing for a race. So keep in mind that these intervals are all about suffering and gaining fitness. Don't worry about your speed, especially when it starts to drop off because of fatigue.

INTERVAL

(5 minutes × 3 minutes × 3)

| | |
|---|---|
| **Total Time** | 45 minutes to 1 hour |
| **Warm-Up** | 15-minute spin |
| **Terrain** | Flat or rolling hills |
| **Training Zone** | 4 |
| **Workout Time** | 21 minutes (15 minutes in zone 4) |
| **Cool-Down** | 10 minutes |

| Effort | Rest |
|---|---|
| 5 minutes | 3 minutes |
| 5 minutes | 3 minutes |
| 5 minutes | Cool-down |

Long Johns are the longest intervals in this chapter. They should be performed at the upper end of zone 4. Maintain the best effort possible for the full 5 minutes. Keep spinning during the 3-minute rest.

Focus on getting into a rhythm during these intervals. You should also work on your position. This will carry over to the time trial workouts in chapter 9. Try to keep your back as flat as possible and pedal in smooth circles.

Vary this workout by doing it with a slightly fast cadence on the first effort, a slow cadence (bigger gear) on the second effort, and a normal cadence on the third. This will work your muscles differently during each cycle and give you something different to focus on during each 5-minute effort.

Performance drops off with increased core body temperature, so you should try to stay as cool as possible. During hard efforts on warm days, periodically pour some water over yourself. This will increase cooling from the wind and give you a little mental boost. For hard interval days, you may want to bring one bottle of rehydration mix and one bottle of plain water for cooling. In desperate times, however, dumping mix over your head won't cause you much harm!

INTERVAL

# UNSTRUCTURED FARTLEK

Never get so caught up in your training that you forget to have a good time. If you're feeling stressed because you didn't stick to your training program, don't waste time fretting about it. Try the Fartlek workout and just have fun! It's never too late to get back on track.

(variable)

| | |
|---|---|
| **Total Time** | 1 hour |
| **Warm-Up** | 10-minute spin |
| **Terrain** | Flat or rolling hills |
| **Training Zone** | 4 to 6 |
| **Workout Time** | 40 minutes |
| **Cool-Down** | 10 minutes |

| Effort | Rest (example) |
|---|---|
| 5 minutes | 2 minutes |
| 1 minute | 3 minutes |
| 45 seconds | 5 minutes |
| 2 minutes | 1 minute |
| Sprint | Cool-down |

The term *fartlek* means "speed play" in Swedish. In simple terms, a fartlek is a variable, continuous interval. In this Unstructured Fartlek workout, you are free to choose whatever pace you like as long as you keep changing things up. For example, you could do a 2-minute interval, followed by a 1-minute rest. Next, perform a 5-minute interval with a 30-second rest. Then switch to a high-speed 15-second burst.

This is a great interval to do with friends. Use road signs or markers to denote the next interval. For example, at the next stop sign, ride hard for 1 minute, recover for 2, and then sprint for the next road sign.

This workout could be a combination of the efforts from the previous intervals in this chapter. There is no right or wrong, just variation. It's like the hippie in interval training—"Just do what you feel is right, man!"

| | |
|---|---|
| **Total Time** | 1 to 1.5 hours |
| **Warm-Up** | 15 minutes |
| **Terrain** | Flat to rolling |
| **Training Zone** | 4 to 6 |
| **Workout Time** | 30 to 60 minutes |
| **Cool-Down** | 15 minutes |

Go to a local bike shop or club in your community and find out when there is a fast training ride. Most areas will have a particular day set aside for a "race ride." If you don't think you're ready for riding in an organized group, then try to get a few friends together to "go hard."

The purpose of the race ride is to force you to ride at someone else's pace. You don't get to predetermine your workout or mentally prepare for set intervals. This is a fast ride that will be different every time. This is different from Canalow, which was described in chapter 6. Canalow is a group ride, but not a race ride. Canalow may include fast sections, such as a climb, but otherwise it's just a group ride. For the Race Ride workout, the riding group should be racing.

I remember being quite nervous before race rides in Davis, California. Over 50 riders would show up and race as if it were the Olympic Games. This was fantastic training and also taught me some basic rules of riding hard in groups. You might be a little scared at first, but you can ease yourself into it. Pretty soon it may become one of the highlights of your training days.

Prepare yourself for the race ride. Cut the packaging tops off of your energy bars or other items you might want to eat. This will make the items easy to access during the heat of battle. The quicker you can get the food into your mouth and get your hands back on the bars, the better off and safer you'll be.

INTERVAL

## Sample Interval Program

| Week | Mon | Tues | Wed | Thurs | Fri | Sat | Sun |
|------|-----|------|-----|-------|-----|-----|-----|
| 1 | Off | Full Recovery Pg. 77 | City Cruise Pg. 61 | Off or gym | Unstructured Fartlek Pg. 84 | Grandma Pg. 64 | Tempo Pg. 65 |
| 2 | Off or gym | Workups Pg. 81 | Tempo Pg. 65 | Coffee Ride Pg. 60 | Off | Race Ride Pg. 85 | Grandma Pg. 64 |
| 3 | Off | Minutemen Pg. 79 | Coffee Ride Pg. 60 | Off or gym | Rave Pg. 68 | Full Recovery Pg. 77 | Big Boy Pg. 63 |
| 4 | Off | Workdowns Pg. 82 | City Cruise Pg. 61 | Off or gym | Holy Roller Pg. 62 | Unstructured Fartlek Pg. 84 | Grandma Pg. 64 |
| 5 | Off | Workdowns Pg. 82 | Off | Long Johns Pg. 83 | Off | Race Ride Pg. 85 | Big Boy Pg. 63 |
| 6 | Off or gym | Double Time Pg. 80 | Tempo Pg. 65 | Off | Rave Pg. 68 | Grandma Pg. 64 | Unstructured Fartlek Pg. 84 |

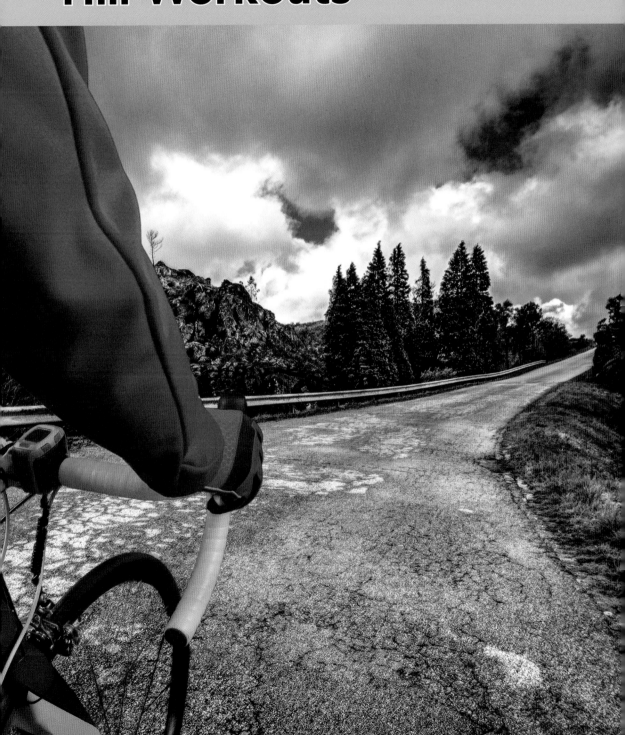

# 8

# Hill Workouts

# Timmy Duggan's View

Timmy Duggan is a member of the Saxo-Tinkoff Pro Cycling Team, a U.S. pro champion (2012), and an Olympian (2012).

Climbing is anything but one dimensional. It seems simple . . . you just have to get to the top, right? But in fact getting to the top of a climb, especially in a race situation, is an extremely dynamic process. Riding alone or in a group, your effort will vary based on the demands of the climb. During a fierce acceleration or extremely steep section, you may have to produce a huge amount of power for a short time, only to recover at your lactate threshold. Whether you are using your diesel power up the 26-kilometer Col de la Croix de Fer in the Alps or sprinting up the steep 1 kilometer of the Cauberg of Amstel Gold, climbing can resemble an explosive 100-meter dash or a grueling but steadier marathon.

In a race, I never get to roll nice and easy into a climb and then race up at my own pace. Often the pace is flat out for several minutes before the climb even starts as everyone fights for positioning. In training, I like to motorpace or do a hard effort into the bottom of the climb to replicate that sensation for the race.

Also, typically the most difficult parts of a climb are the very beginning and the very end. I like to replicate this in training by doing a very hard effort at the bottom of a climb; then I have to do the rest of the climb loaded up from that effort. Over the top, I do another final surge with the effort of the climb weighing heavy in my legs.

The workouts in this chapter definitely reflect the various tools that you need sharpened in order to be an effective climber in any situation. It's all about being able to handle anything that the climb or other riders throw at you while still being able to recover and keep going at a hard pace.

**This** may turn out to be your favorite training chapter in the book. Or maybe you will say just the opposite. Some cyclists are climbers, and some are flatlanders. Even if you are in the latter group, you're going to have to go up every once in a while. If you enjoy climbing, then you'll eat up these workouts.

The climbing workouts focus on three things: (1) lactate threshold, (2) sustained power, and (3) technique. Climbing well requires that you train each aspect. The workouts that follow will help you focus your effort so that you get the most out of your climbing days.

The higher your lactate threshold, the faster you'll be able to ride up a mountain. You want to continue to push your threshold upward toward your maximal heart rate. The higher your threshold, the higher your power output. Your cardiovascular system will deliver sustained energy to your muscles, which in turn will be able to more forcefully contract for an extended period of time.

These workouts will also improve your muscle strength. Climbing is similar to going to a gym for a weight workout. As you climb, you're lifting a weight against gravity. It's the same work you perform when you lift a leg sled against gravity on a gym lifting machine. With repeated hill workouts, your muscles will hypertrophy (grow), gaining strength and power. Couple this with more efficient energy delivery as your threshold increases, and you'll become a climbing machine.

Climbing isn't only about mashing on the pedals for as long and hard as you can. You also need to be efficient. Don't waste energy by flinging your body all over the bike as you grimace with your effort. Try to remain calm on the bike. Keep your shoulders from bouncing and your head from rocking. Apply power throughout the whole rotation of your pedal stroke. Don't expend extra energy by requiring your downstroking leg to lift a non-contributing upstroking leg.

Cyclists should climb in the saddle as much as possible. However, that doesn't mean that it is bad to stand. Sometimes standing is necessary. For example, a steep pitch of the road, a switchback, an acceleration, or even a muscle ache may require you to get out of the saddle. When I'm climbing, I periodically stand just to keep my old bones from feeling too cramped up. Standing mixes up the climb a little and gives my mind a break. This can do wonders when you're putting in a hard effort.

Remember that the days spent climbing are also the days you get to practice your descents. Some of the best climbers in the world have lost bike races because the other guy was better at descents and gained an advantage on the way down. In general, you should descend with your hands in the drops. Keep your eyes down the road so you can plan your path. If you have a chance, watch car or motorcycle racing. Those racers are fantastic at picking the right path to bring them through the apex of a turn.

## Cycling Spotlight

A professional cyclist once told me how to descend fast. He said, "If you want to ride fast, do three things. One, get on my wheel; two, don't touch your brakes; and three, don't freak out." That is easier said than done when you're careening down a hill at 55 mph! You must take the time to learn how to descend. You're not out to win the Tour de France, so take good care of yourself. Work on technique, positioning, and form. Stay comfortable, and enjoy the ride to the bottom.

# QUARTERS

Attack the climb! Be mentally prepared to go up! Think about your training before the ride. Wrap your brain around the fact that you CAN climb and that your fitness will improve with mountain efforts. By not believing in their abilities, many people sabotage their effort before they ever get on the road.

| | |
|---|---|
| **Total Time** | 1 to 1.5 hours |
| **Warm-Up** | 15 minutes |
| **Terrain** | Mountains or hills |
| **Training Zone** | 4 and 5 |
| **Workout Time** | 24 to 66 minutes |
| **Cool-Down** | 10 minutes |

Scope out a good climb in your area. Ideally, it will have a similar grade throughout, but you may have to make do with what's available. The workout is called Quarters because you will divide the climb into four sections, or quarters. Do at least two repeats; you can do more depending on the length of the climb and your fitness level. Each quarter (section) will be a 3-minute interval.

**First climb:**

| | |
|---|---|
| Quarter 1 | Zone 5 |
| Quarter 2 | Zone 4 |
| Quarter 3 | Zone 5 |
| Quarter 4 | Zone 4 |

**Second climb:**

| | |
|---|---|
| Quarter 1 | Zone 4 |
| Quarter 2 | Zone 5 |
| Quarter 3 | Zone 4 |
| Quarter 4 | Zone 5 |

Third climb: Keep alternating as on the previous climbs.

These workouts are difficult because your "recovery" is performed at the level of your LT (zone 4: tempo). You are training your body to cope with all the waste products of the previous effort while still trying to keep a reasonable pace going up the mountain. Fun, fun, fun!

HILL

| | |
|---|---|
| **Total Time** | 50 to 90 minutes |
| **Warm-Up** | 15 minutes |
| **Terrain** | Mountains or hills |
| **Training Zone** | 4 and 5 |
| **Workout Time** | 24 to 66 minutes |
| **Cool-Down** | 15 to 20 minutes |

These rides put you into the hurt cellar. The idea is to train your body to continue to function while you're building up lactic acid. A straight interval involves doing an effort and then recovering before you start the next. Similar to the Quarters workout, Climbing Negatives requires you to recover on the move. After your warm-up, do a 30-second climbing interval in zone 5. You will likely be standing as you accelerate up to speed and then maintain a good effort for 30 seconds. Then sit down and settle into an aggressive zone 4 climb for 5 minutes. Repeat as your fitness allows.

Keep your cadence up while climbing. If you feel yourself start to slow, stand up so you can keep your legs pumping. If you have to accelerate on a climb, you'll be much more responsive if you stand to ramp up your effort.

HILL

# SLOW-RIDER CLIMB

If you are riding in colder weather, especially when climbing, make sure you layer your clothes. Wearing multiple layers is often better than wearing one thick jacket. You'll heat up during your ride up the hill, but you'll need to stop the wind and chill on the way down. By layering, you can unzip and even remove layers as needed. If you get good, you'll be able to do this on the move, but you must be careful. Saving a few seconds isn't worth a crash.

| | |
|---|---|
| **Total Time** | 1 to 1.5 hours |
| **Warm-Up** | 15 minutes |
| **Terrain** | Mountain or hills |
| **Training Zone** | 3 or 4 |
| **Workout Time** | 30 minutes to 1 hour |
| **Cool-Down** | 15 minutes easy with a quick cadence |

Ready to be a powerful climber? Think of Slow-Rider Climb as a climbing-specific weight training workout. This workout is similar to doing repeated, high-volume squats in the gym. The goal is to develop staying power while climbing.

Each interval is 10 minutes long followed by a 5-minute easy spin. If you normally climb with a cadence between 85 and 100 rpm, then the interval should be done between 55 and 65 rpm.

Focus on all aspects of your form while doing these intervals. Think about your back position, your hands on the tops or hoods of your bike, and keeping your body smooth with no bounce. Pedal throughout the complete revolution. Imagine that you are tearing up the most difficult climb you have to do. This interval is not about speed; it's about power and form. Remember, this ride can be rough on your joints, so make sure you ease into it and give yourself plenty of rest and recovery afterward.

| | |
|---|---|
| **Total Time** | 1 to 1.5 hours |
| **Warm-Up** | 15 minutes |
| **Terrain** | Mountains or hills |
| **Training Zone** | 4 |
| **Workout Time** | 30 minutes to 1 hour |
| **Cool-Down** | 15 minutes |

Now for the combination ride. Ride for 10 minutes at a slow cadence, similar to the cadence used in the Slow-Rider Climb workout. Recover for 5 minutes. Then, ride at a fast cadence (115 to 125 rpm) for 10 minutes. Recover for 5 minutes and repeat. These intervals will confuse your muscles a bit, and that is the whole point. Like in all the other workouts, you should focus on your form. You'll get to really know your body sensations when you switch back and forth between super-slow cadence and fast cadence.

Cornering while descending is exhilarating but at the same time nerve racking. As you come into the corner, focus on pushing your foot through the pedal and into the ground on your outside pedal. This will help drive the center of gravity of your bike to the ground and increase your balance and stability.

HILL

# UP–DOWNS

If you need a place to store extra clothing or a raincoat, you can use the second water bottle on your bike. Cut off the top of the bottle and stuff the clothing item inside. Slip the bottle into your bike's second bottle holder, and you have yourself a handy storage container.

| | |
|---|---|
| **Total Time** | 1 to 1.5 hours |
| **Warm-Up** | 15 minutes |
| **Terrain** | Mountain or hills |
| **Training Zone** | 3 |
| **Workout Time** | 30 to 60 minutes |
| **Cool-Down** | 15 minutes |

Start your climb by standing for 2 minutes. Smoothly transition to sitting for 2 more minutes. Continue to switch between sitting and standing every 2 minutes until you reach 10 minutes. Take a break for 5 minutes, riding easy and comfortably. Repeat the interval again. Your fitness level will determine how many intervals you do. You should ride in zone 3, just below your LT. This workout will help improve your transition between sitting and standing. It will also help you create a natural rhythm between sitting and standing when you do longer climbs. Remember, climbing while sitting is efficient, but there will be times (such as increased gradients and surges) when you are required to transition between sitting and standing.

HILL

| | |
|---|---|
| **Total Time** | 45 to 75 minutes |
| **Warm-Up** | 15 minutes |
| **Terrain** | Mountain or hills |
| **Training Zone** | 3 and 5 |
| **Workout Time** | 12 to 45 minutes |
| **Cool-Down** | 15 minutes |

Begin riding at a normal, steady tempo just below your LT (zone 3: tempo). Pretend that you need to close down the gap to another rider or need to put a little distance between you and your riding partner. Execute an acceleration, or jump, and maintain the increased speed for the next 30 seconds (zone 5: super threshold). Slow down to zone 3 for the next minute. Repeat the interval with another 30-second jump. These intervals are 30 seconds on followed by a 1-minute rest. As with all the workouts, your fitness level will dictate the number of efforts. Shoot for 5 to 10, but do more if you're fit. Keep repeating until you feel a significant drop-off in your speed during the jump. These intervals are effective because they simulate race climbing. Watch the races on TV and you'll see riders attack, sit in, and then attack again.

Don't sit upright when you crest the top of a climb. Many riders hit the top and immediately let up on the pedals and rest. But that is just the time you want to distance yourself from your opponent. The moment you crest the summit your speed will rapidly increase, creating an apparently larger gap for anyone following. It will help motivate you and demoralize your opponent. You don't always have to be a nice guy while training!

HILL

# THE CHASER

If possible, avoid braking while zipping through a corner on a descent. Ideally, you should brake before you come into the corner and then glide through smoothly. Obviously, you want to avoid losing traction and sliding out in a corner. When you brake, some of the forces used to keep you from sliding are used in slowing. This increases the likelihood of losing traction. See, your high school physics *is* relevant to your normal life!

| | |
|---|---|
| **Total Time** | 45 minutes to 1.5 hours |
| **Warm-Up** | 15 minutes |
| **Terrain** | Mountain or hills |
| **Training Zone** | 4 and 5 |
| **Workout Time** | 15 to 45 minutes |
| **Cool-Down** | 15 minutes |

If possible, this ride is best done with a training partner. One rider is the rabbit; the other is the hunter. Have your partner start off climbing at tempo (a solid, quick pace, but not completely putting himself in the hurt locker). Allow the partner to gain a gap up the road of about 100 meters (or yards). Now, accelerate and reel the partner in. Close the gap at a crisp pace without burying yourself. (You'll have to keep riding once you catch the rabbit.) Ride at the partner's tempo for the next minute. Then, slowly allow him to pull away again, creating the 100-meter gap. Repeat the process by accelerating and reeling him in once again. You can do all sorts of variations with this ride. Take turns back and forth with your partner on the same day. Or, trade off on different days. One day you work at tempo; the other you work The Chaser.

HILL

| | |
|---|---|
| **Total Time** | 45 minutes to 1.5 hours |
| **Warm-Up** | 15 minutes |
| **Terrain** | Mountain or hills |
| **Training Zone** | 4 |
| **Workout Time** | 15 to 45 minutes |
| **Cool-Down** | 15 minutes |

This is a simple training ride. It is similar to the LT test described in chapter 3. Find a lovely climb, and ride at a solid constant pace. This is about settling into the climb and finding a natural rhythm. You'll have to play with your gearing to find your cadence "sweet spot." Training at tempo will give you confidence when you hit the bottom of a climb. You'll know your limits and the pace that you can sustain for a prolonged period.

When you reach the top of a climb, never stop just over the summit. Keep pedaling another 50 to 100 meters (or yards) to get your momentum started for the downhill. If you are in a competition or trying to get your personal best time on a ride, you'll gain valuable seconds by finishing the climb "just past the climb."

HILL

# RECOVERY CLIMB

Always wear a helmet. Some riders take off their helmets when climbing. Unfortunately, you can crash or be hit even on the uphill. You don't need much forward speed to slam hard into the ground. I've done it myself. My front wheel slipped on some gravel at a switchback, and I did a pile driver into the ground. My helmet broke off of my head, and I didn't even have a headache!

| | |
|---|---|
| **Total Time** | 30 minutes to 1 hour |
| **Warm-Up** | Not necessary |
| **Terrain** | Mountain or hills |
| **Training Zone** | 2 |
| **Workout Time** | 30 minutes to 1 hour |
| **Cool-Down** | Not necessary |

You know you're becoming a mountain goat if you can actually do a recovery ride while climbing. This ride is about spinning easy up a hill. Don't worry about what the speedometer says. This shouldn't be a struggle, so don't choose a climb that's too steep. The road should have a subtle grade that lets your gearing take the effort out of the climb. Chat with a friend to ensure that you're not going too hard. Again, concentrate on your form. Remark to yourself, "Hey, this climbing deal isn't so hard after all."

HILL

## Sample Climbing Program

| Week | Mon | Tues | Wed | Thurs | Fri | Sat | Sun |
|------|-----|------|-----|-------|-----|-----|-----|
| 1 | Off | Quarters Pg. 90 | City Cruise Pg. 61 | Off or gym | Slow Rider Pg. 66 | Grandma Pg. 64 | Tempo Pg. 65 |
| 2 | Off or gym | Up–Downs Pg. 94 | Tempo Pg. 65 | Coffee Ride Pg. 60 | Tempo Pg. 65 | Off | Grandma Pg. 64 |
| 3 | Off or gym | Climbing Negatives Pg. 91 | City Cruise Pg. 61 | Off | Switcher Climb Pg. 93 | Coffee Ride Pg. 60 | Big Boy Pg. 63 |
| 4 | Off | Tempo Pg. 65 | Jumpy Pg. 95 | Off or gym | City Cruise Pg. 61 | Race Ride Pg. 85 | Big Boy Pg. 63 |
| 5 | Off | Quarters Pg. 90 | Rave Pg. 68 | Off or gym | Tempo Pg. 65 | Race Ride Pg. 85 | Grandma Pg. 64 |
| 6 | Off | Jumpy Pg. 95 | Tempo Pg. 65 | Off or gym | Rave Pg. 68 | City Cruise Pg. 61 | Grandma Pg. 64 |

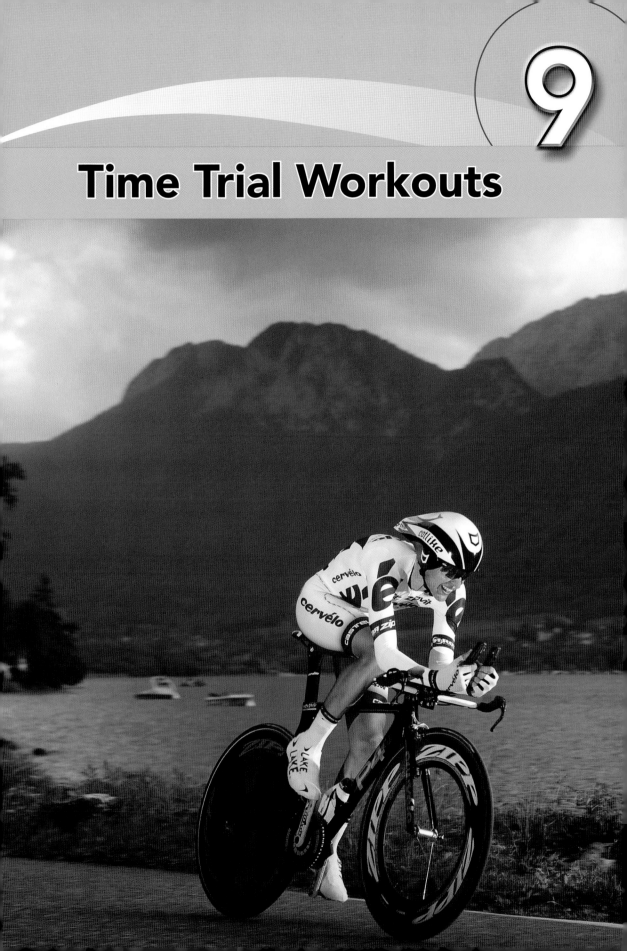

# Time Trial Workouts

# 9

# Alex Howes' View

Alex Howes is a member of the Garmin Sharp Barracuda Pro Cycling Team. He has been the U.S. National Under 23 Road and Criterium Champion and a stage winner at Tour of Utah.

Time trials are rough. There really is no way around it. The saying "It never gets easier; you just go faster" is most appropriate when applied to the discipline of time trials. I have always struggled in the race against the clock. A lightweight, lanky frame and poor flexibility have set me up for less-than-stellar times. However, with attention to detail, hard work, and the proper motivation, the time trial can be one of the most rewarding disciplines in cycling. There are few things more exhilarating than smashing an old personal record time or humming along at high speed under your own power.

Choose a circuit that you can ride on regularly. In your diary, keep track of the various conditions of the ride: wind speed, temperature, and time of year. Then make note of your riding variables. You need to track it all, including body position, head position, and hand position. Pay close attention to your cadence. I shaved more than a minute from my circuit by just changing my head position—no wind tunnel or anything. I had more speed, less average power, and a better time. Put in the work off the bike as well. Improving flexibility in the lower back and hamstrings will go a long way toward improving not only your position and power but your comfort level as well. Pay attention to your equipment. Aero bars and a good set of wheels go a long way, but make sure you put in the necessary time dialing in your position so that you feel aerodynamic and comfortable. You want to have your mind focused on the effort and not the funky aero bars or the deep dish wheel getting slapped around by the wind. If you make only one upgrade to your bike, make sure you have a saddle you feel comfortable on. If you are dreading getting on your bike because your butt hurts or you cannot get into a low position because you are sitting on a rock, your times will suffer immensely.

Perhaps the most important thing for me when time trialing is finding the motivation to suffer. To do a great time trial, you must literally be right on the edge the whole time. Losing focus for just a few minutes is usually the difference between winning and losing. I have seen riders do nearly everything to try to find that last 1 percent of motivation to go harder. Meditation, reading break-up letters from exes, thinking about the boss who will not cut you any slack—those are all good tactics for finding that edge. Some riders make a point of thinking about why they are riding. Riding or racing for a charity or fundraiser always seems to elevate people's performance. Others think about whom they are riding for by racing with a picture of their family tucked away in their helmet or under their saddle. I read a few lines from *The Way of the Samurai* before important events. Do whatever it takes.

**Time** trialing has become all the rage, and for good reason. It is a great way to monitor your progress, compete against yourself, and focus on technical aspects of riding a bike. Some cyclists only compete in time trials. They don't like the risks and direct competition of criteriums and road racing, but they find the race against the clock to be the perfect avenue to satisfy the racer within. Clubs all over are putting on time trial events, increasing the accessibility to all levels of riders. Even if you don't compete, all you need is a stopwatch to monitor your progress and fitness.

Whether you plan on competing in an organized TT event or not, TT training should be a part of every well-rounded training program. Specialized TT training improves endurance, power, and mental toughness. It also helps you gain an understanding of aerodynamics and efficiency. Regardless of your goal, including these workouts in your training program will definitely up your game.

In 1989, Greg LeMond won the Tour de France by only 8 seconds over Laurent Fignon. Only 8 seconds! The Tour de France that year was 21 stages, 2,041 miles long, and it all came down to a measly 8 seconds. LeMond won the race on the final stage, an individual TT of 15.5 miles. LeMond was 50 seconds down, and most people thought that it was far too much time to make up over such a short distance. Always the innovator, Greg LeMond used aerobars for the first time in the event. Fignon did not. The aerodynamic efficiency of the aerobar brought Greg LeMond to the pinnacle of his sport. He obliterated his competitors, in large part because of his amazing physiology, but also because of the aerodynamic advantage of the aerobar. If you like bike racing and have never seen the 1989 Tour de France, then make a night of it and watch the video. It is a fantastic and exciting race. (While you're at it, you could also watch the 1989 World Championship, which may be my favorite race of all time!)

This story about Greg LeMond and aerobars doesn't mean that you should feel obligated to go out and spend money on aerodynamic equipment. Rather, it points out the importance of maintaining an efficient position on the bike. Whether you use aerobars, disc wheels, or skin suits—or just go out and ride in shorts and a T-shirt—you should always think about how much the wind is hindering your progress. Pay attention to the details of your position on the bike. When riding, try to minimize your impact with the wind. Your position is a trade-off between aerodynamics, comfort, and the ability to deliver power to the cranks. All three factors need to be addressed when setting up your bicycle. Chapter 14 provides information that will give you a good start on finding the best position, but that will only set you on the right path. By practicing the TT, you'll be able to see real changes in your efficiency and power with training. Pay attention to the plane of your body and how it comes in contact with the wind as you ride. Make small adjustments during your training rides to see if anything works better than your current setup.

## Cycling Spotlight

You don't have to be a racer to benefit from TT training. This type of training is good for all cyclists. It increases your LT and leg strength, makes you mentally tough, and hones in correct riding form. TT training is also effective because riding against the clock keeps you honest. One aspect of the RACE training philosophy is accountability. The clock keeps you accountable. Go to the same course and ride it periodically. Try to keep the conditions consistent. The numbers won't lie. If you are consistently training, you'll definitely see periodic improvements, and that's the whole purpose of your training: to improve, ride faster, and obtain your goals! Performing TT workouts is hard work, but the benefits will be obvious as your fitness continues to improve.

Focus on your cadence and pedal stroke. Make sure you're applying smooth power. You can listen to the revolutions as you ride. Ideally, you'd like to hear a steady hum rather than a whaa-whaa-whaa with each pedal downstroke. Try to pedal consistent circles, applying power throughout the revolution as best you can. Experiment with a slightly faster and slower cadence than you normally use in order to see if it changes your speed, leg burn, breathing, or RPE.

| | |
|---|---|
| **Total Time** | 45 minutes to 1 hour |
| **Warm-Up** | 10 minutes |
| **Terrain** | Flat |
| **Training Zone** | 3 |
| **Workout Time** | 27 to 45 minutes |
| **Cool-Down** | 10 minutes |

Most people favor one leg over the other. This workout is designed to train each leg individually. Your weak leg won't be able to run or hide any longer! Each interval trains only one leg at a time. Complete a full and solid pedal stroke using only your right leg. Your left leg is catching a free ride, rotating without effort as your right leg does all the work. Concentrate on providing consistent power throughout the pedal stroke of the leg doing the interval. After 3 minutes, switch immediately to the other leg. Each interval set is a total of 6 minutes. When you complete a 3-minute cycle with each leg, begin your rest phase. Pedal equally at an easy spin with both legs for 3 minutes. Repeat the entire cycle as many times as your fitness allows.

Be comfortable off the bike. If you work hard while riding, work hard at being comfortable. As soon as you're cleaned up after your ride, put on comfortable clothes. Get out of your wet shorts and jersey. You can make it a personal tradition—favorite sweatpants, sweat top, and shoes for lounging.

TIME TRIAL

Always ride with some sort of identification and emergency contact information. Put your contact information in your saddlebag. You can purchase professionally made items such as dog tags or bracelets (e.g. Road ID). Let's hope that you never crash, but it is better to be safe than sorry.

| | |
|---|---|
| **Total Time** | 50 to 70 minutes |
| **Warm-Up** | 15 minutes |
| **Terrain** | Flat |
| **Training Zone** | 3 |
| **Workout Time** | 20 to 40 minutes |
| **Cool-Down** | 15 minutes |

Form, form, form. This entire workout is more about form than fitness (but you'll get some of that as well). The object of this workout is to dial in your perfect position. You want to feel comfortable, strong, and FAST. Imagine riding a TT for the gold medal. That would define a 100 percent TT effort. This training ride should be at 70 to 80 percent effort. The reduced wattage lets you focus on your form (rather than focus only on how much you are suffering). Follow the advice of Alex Howes. Keep notes and ride the same course on multiple training days. Find out what works and what doesn't. Change only one aspect at a time so you get a clear picture of how it affects your performance. Your diary will be invaluable for comparison.

TIME TRIAL

| | |
|---|---|
| **Total Time** | 1 to 1.5 hours |
| **Warm-Up** | 15 minutes |
| **Terrain** | Flat |
| **Training Zone** | 4 |
| **Workout Time** | 20 to 40 minutes |
| **Cool-Down** | 15 minutes |

Get ready to make your legs and back burn! These are power intervals in your TT position. After you're good and warm, perform a 10-minute TT power interval. Your cadence should be about 10 to 15 percent slower than your optimal speed. (By doing the Practice Makes Perfect workout, you should have a good idea of your proper cadence.) If you ideally ride a TT with an rpm of 100, you should ride this workout at 85 to 90. Keep your speed up and work hard. You should feel very spent at the end of 10 minutes. Take a 5-minute rest and then repeat. Do at least two intervals (do more if you can tolerate it). Turning a big gear in your TT position will help you develop raw power. It's similar to a baseball player swinging two baseball bats before going to the plate. When you perform at a normal cadence, you'll feel strong and fast.

Be determined. Before you start any ride or workout, review your goals. Prepare yourself mentally and be determined to give 100 percent effort. I was talking with David Millar after he won stage 12 in the 2012 Tour de France. He said, "I was determined. I was going to win." Once he was in the breakaway, he never had doubts or thought of anything less than victory. "I knew I had to win!"

TIME TRIAL

# SPINNAGE

A cyclist is always going to have aches and pains while training. Part of pushing your body hard is the resultant adaptation. Sometimes your body will rebel a bit and push back in the form of aching muscles, colds, and fatigue. That is all part of the game. Don't become discouraged. Just take good care of yourself and work the problem until you've recovered.

| | |
|---|---|
| **Total Time** | 1 to 1.5 hours |
| **Warm-Up** | 15 minutes |
| **Terrain** | Flat or slightly downhill |
| **Training Zone** | 3 |
| **Workout Time** | 20 to 40 minutes |
| **Cool-Down** | 15 minutes |

This workout is similar to Powerhouse but on the other extreme. For this training, after you're warm, ride a 10 minute TT with a faster cadence than normal. Keep your RPM 10 to 15 percent above normal. It is helpful to perform this workout on a slight downhill. This workout is more about smooth pedaling circles and form than pure cardio work. You need to look good on the bike, so focus on each of the points of contact. Focus on a flat back, no bounce, and good leg speed. Think of being majestic and controlled on your bike.

TIME TRIAL

| | |
|---|---|
| **Total Time** | 50 to 70 minutes |
| **Warm-Up** | 15 minutes |
| **Terrain** | Flat |
| **Training Zone** | 4 or 5 |
| **Workout Time** | 20 to 40 minutes |
| **Cool-Down** | 15 minutes |

Watch it all come together. This is your TT test. See how fast you can ride a 20- to 40-minute individual TT. This workout is your benchmark. You'll continually come back to the same course to see your improvements. This is where you'll determine if the items you perfected during the Practice Makes Perfect workouts change your performance when you ride full gas. Act as if this is a world championship performance. Leading up to this training day, you should mentally prepare yourself and fuel up. No excuses. Just get out there and ride as fast as you can. Ride like the wind (or in the world of the cyclist, into the wind!).

You can use one of your riding partners to stabilize yourself on a ride. If you need to take your attention away from the road momentarily, hold the shoulder of your riding partner. This will keep you moving in a straight line and will add stability. It is a great technique to use while riding in a pack (when you need to mind your space). As always, practice this skill carefully.

TIME TRIAL

# ENOUGH IS ENOUGH

Caffeine acts as a stimulant and a diuretic (it makes you pee). Although you might want the first attribute on the ride, you definitely don't want the second. Be aware that the more caffeine you take in—either through coffee, energy drinks, or loaded gels—the more you'll have to urinate. This can add to potential dehydration, not to mention the annoyance of having to stop on a ride to heed the call of nature.

| | |
|---|---|
| **Total Time** | 50 to 70 minutes |
| **Warm-Up** | 15 minutes |
| **Terrain** | Flat |
| **Training Zone** | 5 |
| **Workout Time** | 20 to 40 minutes |
| **Cool-Down** | 15 minutes |

You're going to love this one . . . NOT! This ride will put you into the hurt cave without a flashlight. Start off by riding a fast 5-minute TT. This should be at a much higher pace than your normal TT workouts. Immediately after the 5 minutes, slow down (just a bit) and try to get into a rhythm at your normal TT speed. Hold this for as long as possible. Depending on your fitness level, this may be 10 to 30 minutes. The idea is to put you in debt and force you to continue to ride. Your body will be doing all it can to keep up with the energy demands and waste products of your workout. It's like tying one hand behind a boxer's back. You will suffer the entire workout, trying to dig yourself out of the hole you created with the first 5 minutes of the workout.

TIME TRIAL

| | |
|---|---|
| **Total Time** | 45 to 50 minutes |
| **Warm-Up** | 15 minutes |
| **Terrain** | Flat |
| **Training Zone** | 5 |
| **Workout Time** | 20 to 40 minutes |
| **Cool-Down** | 15 minutes |

This is similar to your LT test, but now you're using it as a straight-up workout. This TT interval starts out at a leisurely pace. Try to keep your cadence fairly constant. Every 2 minutes, increase your speed by 1 mph. Maintain your form, even when you feel as though the oxygen content in the atmosphere has suddenly plummeted. It may take a workout or two for you to find the ideal starting speed. If you enjoy this workout, then (1) you're crazy, and (2) you can try variations. Increase your speed every 30 seconds, or increase your speed every 3 minutes. The first will give you a high-speed, high-energy workout, while the latter will prolong the suffering with a slow grind to exhaustion.

If your derailleur breaks on a ride, you can turn your bike into a single speed by using your chain tool. Disconnect the chain. Reroute the chain directly around the front and rear chainring, avoiding the derailleur altogether. Reconnect the chain, taking out the extra tension. You should be able to ride without a problem. Keep in mind that you cannot shift EITHER the front or rear chainrings.

TIME TRIAL

# UNDONE

Draw the imprint of the cleat on the bottom of your shoe with a permanent marker so you know its exact position if it comes loose. You can also make a small mark in your seat tube where it enters the downtube. Again, this way if it comes loose you'll know the exact height of your saddle. Your knees will be grateful.

| | |
|---|---|
| **Total Time** | 45 to 50 minutes |
| **Warm-Up** | 15 minutes of spinning, including a single 1-minute hard interval |
| **Terrain** | Flat |
| **Training Zone** | 4 |
| **Workout Time** | 20 to 40 minutes |
| **Cool-Down** | 15 minutes |

This is the opposite of Windup. You should perform Windup at least once before trying Undone so you have an idea of your maximal TT speed. The warm-up is important for this one. About 10 minutes into your warm-up, you should do a hard 1-minute interval to loosen up. Then spin for 4 to 5 minutes before starting the Undone workout. Start the workout by slowly increasing your speed to your maximal TT velocity. Hold this for 2 minutes and then decrease your speed by 1 mph. Maintain this new speed for 2 more minutes and then decrease it once again by 1 mph. Continue to do this until you're recovered and riding easy.

## Sample Time Trial Program

| Week | Mon | Tues | Wed | Thurs | Fri | Sat | Sun |
|------|-----|------|-----|-------|-----|-----|-----|
| 1 | Pedal to the Metal Pg. 109 | Coffee Ride Pg. 60 | Tempo Pg. 65 | Off or gym | Single Leg Pg. 105 | Big Boy Pg. 65 | Unstructured Fartlek Pg. 84 |
| 2 | Practice Makes Perfect Pg. 106 | Off | Powerhouse Pg. 107 | Off | Tempo Pg. 65 | Coffee Ride Pg. 60 | Tempo Pg. 65 |
| 3 | Off or gym | Enough Is Enough Pg. 110 | Tempo Pg. 65 | Off | Rave Pg. 68 | Big Boy Pg. 63 | Single Leg Pg. 105 |
| 4 | Off | Practice Makes Perfect Pg. 106 | City Cruise Pg. 61 | Off or gym | Spinnage Pg. 108 | Race Ride Pg. 85 | Grandma Pg. 64 |
| 5 | Off | Windup Pg. 111 | Off or gym | Tempo Pg. 65 | Undone Pg. 112 | City Cruise Pg. 61 | Big Boy Pg. 63 |
| 6 | Off | Powerhouse Pg. 107 | Off or gym | Practice Makes Perfect Pg. 106 | City Cruise Pg. 61 | Pedal to the Metal Pg. 109 | Off |

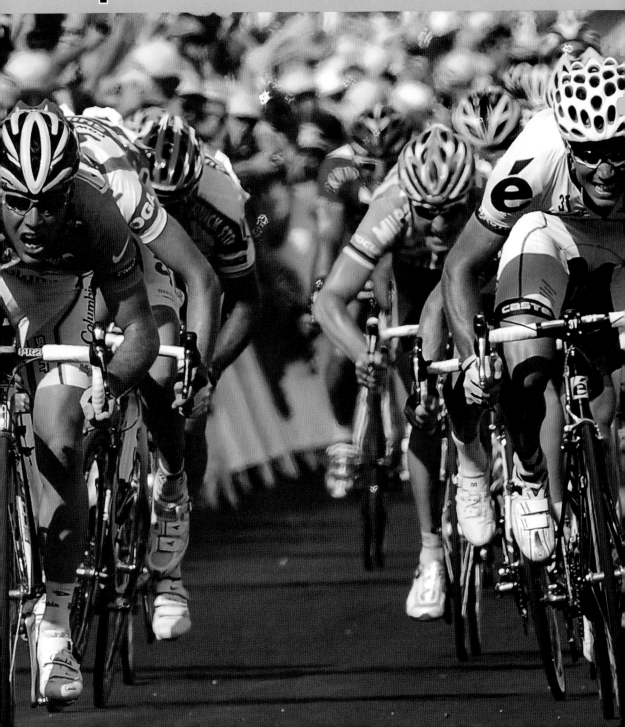

# 10

# Sprint Workouts

# Tyler Farrar's View

Tyler Farrar is a member of Team Garmin-Sharp-Barracuda. He has won stages in the Tour de France, Giro di Italia, and Vuelta a Espana and is also an Olympian.

For me, the most important preparation is replicating the race. In my training, I attempt to match my race conditions. I need to practice with the same speed and fatigue that I experience at the end of a tough race. With your training, you should always try to replicate the way you want to perform your goal.

All the workouts in the book will help you develop speed and power. In addition, there are a few that I personally use to dial in my training. If I have access to motorpacing, I'll do 4-kilometer lead-outs, approaching 50 to 65 kpm. I come around with about 300 meters to go. I like to be in the "red" before I sprint. You have to get your legs loaded up with lactate to simulate how you really feel in a race.

If I'm not motorpacing, I like to do three sets of three sprints, each being 10-second accelerations in an easy gear (I actually spin out). I rest for 10 minutes and then perform three normal sprints—just the way I would in a race. I rest for another 10 minutes before performing three sprints from standing in my 53 × 11 gearing. It's like weightlifting on my bike!

I always make my training a little harder than it has to be. For example, if I'm comfortable sprinting 250 meters in a race, I always train to sprint 300. Knowing that I've put the training in gives me confidence when we're barreling down the finishing stretch.

If I've done it right and come into the sprint finish of a race in top form, I feel as if time slows down. The last 5 kilometers seem like an eternity. I'm so amped and nervous that the last 2 kilometers seem to take even longer. I don't even feel my legs when I wind up to full speed. If the race seems to get ahead of me and I feel as though I'm behind the eight ball, then I know that I don't have "good" legs.

There's nothing better than winning a race! Set your goal, train for it, and then feel confident that it is in your grasp. My favorite time is the few moments right after I cross the line. The media, officials, teammates, and soigneurs still haven't caught me; and I have a brief few moments to myself. I think about all the training and effort, and I feel the relief, gratification, and excitement of the win!

**Sprinters** have to be a little bit insane. Every time I'm working at a bike race and it comes down to a sprint finish, my heart rate starts to climb. One of our team directors once asked me if it's normal to get sweaty palms during the final moments of a bike race. He kept wiping his hands on his pants as our car raced to keep up with the lead riders as they tore up the last few kilometers before the finishing stretch.

If you've ever seen a race in person, you will appreciate the velocity at which the riders cross the line. Sprinters start racing for position during the last 5 to 10 kilometers (3.1 to 6.2 miles) of the race, usually having teammates sacrifice any remaining energy to move them exactly where they want to be when the final kilometer sign passes overhead. They then put their trust in a reliable lead-out rider who brings them up to nearly top speed. With only a few hundred meters remaining, the sprinter takes flight. All the sprinter's might and energy are harnessed to achieve maximal speed. The sprinter truly finds another gear that only a select few riders ever experience.

Sprinters are amazing specimens. They possess raw power, incredible leg speed, and a sense that there is no way they can die today! Only very few can ever hope to race with that kind of speed and voracity. But, that doesn't mean that every bike rider shouldn't practice the skills needed for a sprint. Part of being a complete rider is knowing how to sprint and having the confidence to mash on your pedals with all your might. Regardless of your goals or training aspirations, you should feel comfortable winding your bike up to speed—with your hands in the drops of the handlebars and with your eyes ahead focused on the prize (even if the prize is a city limit sign).

Sprint training is valuable, and this chapter will help you become a better rider even if you never plan on contesting a sprint at the end of a bike race. The workouts in this chapter are designed to give you power, leg speed, and the ability to rev the tachometer while riding. All of this will translate to other aspects of your riding. By working the high end of your power output and speed, you'll improve the efficiency of your energy delivery system, the network of vascular supply to your muscles, and the contractile force and groupings of your muscle fibers. This will pay dividends when riding at tempo, performing a time trial, climbing a hill, or just seeing how close you can push a ride to the limit.

These workouts will also give you confidence on the bike. You'll start to feel comfortable when your hands are in the handlebar drops and you are giving a powerful effort. Spending time straining for top speed will teach you bike-handling skills and the limits of your riding machine. To be a performance cyclist, you need to become totally comfortable with all aspects of your riding—climbing, descending, cornering, sprinting, and prolonged training rides. By focusing on all of these aspects individually, you will become the best performance cyclist possible.

Winding your bike up to your maximal speed requires more than stomping on the pedals. You need to coordinate your entire body in order to deliver smooth and consistent power to the drivetrain. As with all the workouts in this book, you must pay close attention to your form. You need to focus on distributing all the power from your core, hips, and legs into the cranks. This starts with a solid connection to the bike. When you sprint, keep your hands in the drops and stand out of the saddle. Keep a slight bend in your arms and lean forward with your chest parallel to the top tube. Make sure your feet are secure in stiff shoes and that the shoes connect solidly to the pedals.

Chapter 14 discusses proper pedaling motion. To get maximal power during a sprint, you'll have to apply torque throughout the pedal stroke. Don't waste any part of the crank rotation. Avoid just thrusting down on the pedals as hard as you possibly can.

Keep your bike under control. Don't let it flail about or move beyond reason. Every movement uses energy and decreases efficiency. Keep your body aligned over the midline of the bike, and don't let your head and neck swing around like a serpent. These workouts will test the limit of both you and your machine. You'll get a feel for a stiff versus a soft bike because during a maximal effort, you'll torque the entire frame.

Finally, get ready to enjoy! Speed workouts are difficult but fun. The workouts are different than your other interval training, and riding your bike fast is downright exhilarating. If you're not a natural born sprinter, then you'll get a lot of bang for your buck with these workouts. You can make the most of your speed training when these interval days are worked into your overall program.

## Cycling Spotlight

In the world of cycling, there is a clear delineation between climbers and sprinters. Sprinters are bigger and stronger, and they develop more sheer power. Climbers are slight, wispy, and smaller. Each group is adapted to their specialized role. Sprinters fight against wind resistance, rolling resistance, and usually only a relatively small amount of gravity (because the majority of sprints are relatively flat). Their increased size allows them to generate a large amount of power with only a marginal expense of frontal wind resistance. However, if you start increasing the incline, the extra mass has a much more profound effect on effort. Power-to-weight ratio becomes much more important than maximal power output alone. That is why climbers are usually small. They can still generate big power, but they don't have to lift as much weight up the climb.

| | |
|---|---|
| **Total Time** | Variable |
| **Warm-Up** | 15 minutes |
| **Terrain** | Flat |
| **Training Zone** | 3 |
| **Workout Time** | 6 minutes (interspersed throughout the ride) |
| **Cool-Down** | 15 minutes |

A speed sandwich is more a technique than an actual training ride. It's described here as an individual workout, but you can incorporate the technique into any of your other training rides.

A Speed Sandwich training ride consists of six repetitions of increased speed performed at various times during a ride that is mostly done in zone 3. Position your hands in the handlebar drops. While in the small front chainring, ride on a flat clear road; slowly increase your cadence while sitting. It should take you about 10 to 15 seconds to reach your maximal leg speed. Maintain your peak rpm for a few seconds and then slowly start to decrease your leg speed until you reach your starting cadence. These should be done as smoothly as possible. Avoid having your butt bounce up and down on the saddle. This is all about fluidity and leg speed. Try to press the limit and extend your rpm potential.

To gain the most power, you should do sprints out of the saddle with your hands in the drops. Squeeze the bars hard to help drive the pedals. Avoid shifting or needing to shift during a true sprint. You'll lose far too much time.

SPRINT

# SIGNS (SPRINTS)

If you're feeling fatigued after your rides, try wearing compression socks or tights. This can be especially helpful if you need to go back to work or sit for considerable periods of time. You can purchase these items in running and cycling shops as well as online. (I've used 2XU compression socks, and they work great.)

| | |
|---|---|
| **Total Time** | 1 hour |
| **Warm-Up** | 15 minutes |
| **Terrain** | Flat |
| **Training Zone** | 6 |
| **Workout Time** | 6 minutes (interspersed throughout the ride) |
| **Cool-Down** | 15 minutes |

This might sound oversimplified and obvious, but there is no way to get better at sprinting without actually doing sprints. The purpose of this training ride is to get you out there actually sprinting.

After warm-up, prepare yourself for some sprinting! You'll do these standing with your hands in the drops and with the chain on the "big ring." Every 3 minutes, pick a road sign off in the distance about 200 meters (600 to 700 feet) away. Rev up your sprint from a normal cruise speed until you're giving your maximal effort. Race until you cross the line. Recover with an easy spin until you feel ready to give your maximal effort again. Repeat the process throughout the ride for a total of six sprints. Each time, pretend that you're in a final sprint in the Tour de France.

SPRINT

120

| | |
|---|---|
| **Total Time** | 1 hour |
| **Warm-Up** | 15 minutes |
| **Terrain** | Mild downhill grade |
| **Training Zone** | 5 |
| **Workout Time** | 10 minutes (interspersed throughout the ride) |
| **Cool-Down** | 15 minutes |

Downhill sprints will train your leg speed. Because you won't have so much resistance, you'll get your bike up to a higher speed on the final approach to the finish line. You should still commit fully to the effort, even though you have a slight downhill.

Perform these sprints standing with your hands in the drops. Ride on a gradual descent, nothing very steep. Concentrate on having good form and keeping your bike under control. Wind up slowly and smoothly. Make sure you don't shy away from giving your maximal effort. You should "spin out" your gearing—meaning that you can't find any more "bite" on the pedals—distributing power from your legs to the cranks. You'll need to shift, but there isn't another option. You'll be in the big front chainring and the smallest rear ring.

Never give up! It sounds cliché, but it is true. Just yesterday, I was following Tyler Farrar in the Tour de France. He had been dropped on the first climb and was in jeopardy of falling so far behind that he would be eliminated by the time cut. I thought he'd never make it as he struggled, against all hope, up the climb. He never gave up, just kept suffering and pushing. Remarkably, after the descent, the peloton slowed, and Tyler was able to regain contact. He ended up finishing the stage and competing for the rest of the sprints in the Tour.

SPRINT

Here's a quick fix! If you damage part of the sidewall on a tire, you can do a quick patch with a dollar bill. Take off the tire. Fold up the dollar bill so that its shape covers the tear and place it inside the tire. Replace the tube and then the wheel. When the tube inflates, the dollar will act as a temporary sidewall.

| | |
|---|---|
| **Total Time** | 1 hour |
| **Warm-Up** | 15 minutes |
| **Terrain** | Mild uphill grade |
| **Training Zone** | 6 |
| **Workout Time** | 4 to 6 minutes (interspersed throughout the ride) |
| **Cool-Down** | 15 minutes |

These efforts demand maximal power. When you did the downhill sprints, you practiced the bread and butter of sprinting—leg speed. Now you're going to practice the other key component—straight-up power!

Uphill sprints are self-explanatory. Do 4 to 6 maximal sprints of 150 meters (about 500 feet) while riding up a slight uphill grade. Stand with your hands in the drops. Make sure the hill is gradual; you still need to be able to truly sprint. It is fine if you want to repeat the same stretch of road by coming down the grade (recovering) after each sprint. Doing the same sprint multiple times is sometimes helpful because you get a real sense for how you feel at the different distances from the finish. At 100 meters to go, you'll feel quite different than at 20 meters to go. Learn how your body is responding to such an extreme effort.

SPRINT

| | |
|---|---|
| **Total Time** | 1 hour |
| **Warm-Up** | 15 minutes |
| **Terrain** | Flat |
| **Training Zone** | 3 |
| **Workout Time** | 10 minutes (interspersed throughout the ride) |
| **Cool-Down** | 15 minutes |

Similar to the Speed Sandwiches, you can intersperse the Coaster technique while doing other training rides. It's nice to mix things up when you're on a long base-training ride.

A Coaster is essentially a sprint in the little front chainring. Position your body for a normal sprint—hands in drops, standing on the pedals. Wind up your sprint, but keep the gearing easy. You should "spin out" far before you feel there is no more power left in your legs. Do at least 10 Coasters during this training ride. The remainder of the ride is spent in zone 2 or 3.

Always bring a phone along when you ride. Put it in a plastic bag to keep it from getting wet from sweat and humidity in your pocket. I've been stranded a few times (because I'm a slow learner), and if I had a phone, those moments of my life would have been markedly less frustrating.

SPRINT

# QUICKIES

Keep a 20-dollar bill inside the end of your handlebar. Unplug the cap, and slide in the money. This is a great permanent hiding spot for some emergency cash. If you break down or find yourself stranded, you'll be glad when you remember that you've stored some money in your handlebar.

| | |
|---|---|
| **Total Time** | 1 hour |
| **Warm-Up** | 15 minutes |
| **Terrain** | Flat |
| **Training Zone** | 5 |
| **Workout Time** | 25 minutes |
| **Cool-Down** | 15 minutes |

Quickies are commonly done by track and field athletes. They can be adapted to be done on your bike. These intervals are sprints that turn on and off in rapid succession. Perform the interval in your big chainring. Give a full sprinting effort for 3 to 5 seconds. Then turn off the power but keep the legs spinning for another 3 to 5 seconds. You can sit down during the "off" phase. Again, stand up and go full gas with a maximal effort for another 3 to 5 seconds. Continue to go back and forth for a total of five cycles of on–off. Take a 5-minute break and then do the sequence a total of 5 or 6 times.

> 5 seconds on, 5 seconds off (spinning)
> 5 seconds on, 5 seconds off (spinning)
> 5 seconds on, 5 seconds off (spinning)
> 5 seconds on, 5 seconds off (spinning)
> 5 seconds on, 5-minute rest
>
> Repeat × 5

The idea behind this workout is to give you explosive "snap." You'll work on your ability to do quick and powerful bursts on your bike. You never know when you'll need a burst of acceleration. It might win you a race or even save your life if you have to avoid an unexpected hazard.

| | |
|---|---|
| **Total Time** | 50 minutes to 1 hour |
| **Warm-Up** | 20 minutes |
| **Terrain** | Flat |
| **Training Zone** | 6 |
| **Workout Time** | 15 to 20 minutes |
| **Cool-Down** | 15 minutes |

In this workout, you'll be doing a series of sprints with each successive sprint in a slightly easier gear. Start in your big front chainring and smallest rear chainring (most difficult gear). Start from a very slow cadence and gradually wind up your rpm until you are at a maximal sprint. Maintain your maximal speed for at least 3 to 5 seconds. Take a rest until recovered. Repeat again, but this time shift the rear derailleur twice so you are now two rings away from the smallest ring (in the rear). Perform the same windup and maximal sprint. The exact gearing isn't important. Just make sure you are in a slightly easier gear for each successive sprint.

**Example:**

Sprint in the 52 × 12 gearing, rest
Sprint in the 52 × 14 gearing, rest
Sprint in the 52 × 16 gearing, rest
Sprint in the 52 × 18 gearing, rest
Sprint in the 52 × 21 gearing, rest

Always prepare your postride food before you go out on your ride. There is nothing worse than coming inside after your ride and then mulling around the kitchen trying to find something to eat. If you can plan your after-ride meal before you go, your glucose-deprived body will thank you when you get back.

SPRINT

125

# PACELINE SPEED

Always look out for the riders behind you. When you are at the front of the paceline, those riders are your responsibility. They can't see the road the way you can, so don't lead them astray. If you see debris or rubbish in the road, point it out with your hand. The riders will know to stay on line with your wheel so they don't hit anything.

| | |
|---|---|
| **Total Time** | 45 to 60 minutes |
| **Warm-Up** | 10 minutes |
| **Terrain** | Flat |
| **Training Zone** | 4 |
| **Workout Time** | 15 minutes |
| **Cool-Down** | 10 minutes |

This is a variation on riding in a paceline or behind another rider. In general, when you ride in a paceline, you have one rider in front of you and one behind you. You need to keep your riding as smooth as possible so your bike doesn't jerk about or change speeds. In a paceline, riders should also normally ride in a slightly bigger (harder) gear than when riding solo in order to help take away some of the variation in speed. In this exercise, however, we're throwing that thought out the window.

You can do this workout with as few as one other rider, or you can do it behind a moped or scooter. Let your training partner know the plan. Ride in the slipstream in a smaller gear than normal. Keep your cadence greater than 110 rpm. Focus on keeping your butt down with no bounce. Try to apply consistent power through the entire revolution. At the end of each interval, sprint around the rider in front of you.

Do at least three 5-minute intervals with your high cadence. Rest for at least 5 minutes between each set. This exercise takes concentration because you really need to think about your form. High-cadence training will not only help you enhance your leg speed, but it will also increase your efficiency and form.

| | |
|---|---|
| **Total Time** | Variable |
| **Warm-Up** | 15 minutes |
| **Terrain** | Variable |
| **Training Zone** | 6 |
| **Workout Time** | Variable (interspersed throughout the ride) |
| **Cool-Down** | 15 minutes |

This is more of a fun training ride idea than a true separate workout. Set up five different points of the ride that will represent sprint finishes. Challenge your friends to sprint finishes. Make it worth your while by betting something—such as pizza, coffee, or beer!

Another variation is to use timing challenges. Pick out a few time points along the ride, such as 20 minutes, 30 minutes, and 40 minutes. Both riders synchronize their computers or watches at the beginning of the ride. At each of those points, whoever is ahead of the other gets a point. The rider with the most points at the end of the ride has to pay up. This is fun because you can use any kind of strategy to get ahead. Maybe it will be a sprint in the last minute, or maybe one of you will slowly start to pick up the pace with 5 minutes to go in hopes of dropping your partner before the time finish. Play with this workout and have fun!

If you are on the road during a cold day and you have to descend, you can use newspaper to help create a barrier between your torso and the wind. Lay out the paper inside your jersey, across your chest and abdomen. This is an old (and current) racing trick. Watch a video of a racer in the Giro coming over the top of a mountain pass, and you'll likely see the racer grab a paper and stuff it in his shirt. This might sound like an old wives' tale, but it works!

SPRINT

## Sample Sprint Program

| Week | Mon | Tues | Wed | Thurs | Fri | Sat | Sun |
|------|-----|------|-----|-------|-----|-----|-----|
| 1 | Off | Uphill Sprints Pg. 122 | Speed Sandwiches Pg. 119 | Off or gym | Signs Pg. 120 | Race Ride Pg. 85 | Coffee Ride Pg. 60 |
| 2 | Off | Uphill Sprints Pg. 122 | On–Offs Pg. 78 | Tempo Pg. 65 | Challenge Pg. 127 | Big Boy Pg. 63 / Coasters Pg. 123 | Rave Pg. 68 |
| 3 | Off or gym | Downhill Sprints Pg. 121 | Speed Sandwiches Pg. 119 | Off | Rave Pg. 68 | Tempo Pg. 65 | Grandma Pg. 64 |
| 4 | Off | Spent Pg. 125 | On–Offs Pg. 78 | Off or gym | Challenge Pg. 127 | Big Boy Pg. 63 / Coasters Pg. 123 | Rave Pg. 68 |
| 5 | Off | Uphill Sprints Pg. 122 | Speed Sandwiches Pg. 119 | Off or gym | Tempo Pg. 65 | Race Ride Pg. 85 | Grandma Pg. 64 |
| 6 | Off | Spent Pg. 125 | On–Offs Pg. 78 | Off or gym | Tempo Pg. 65 | Big Boy Pg. 63 | Spinnage Pg. 108 |

# 11

# Stationary Bike Workouts

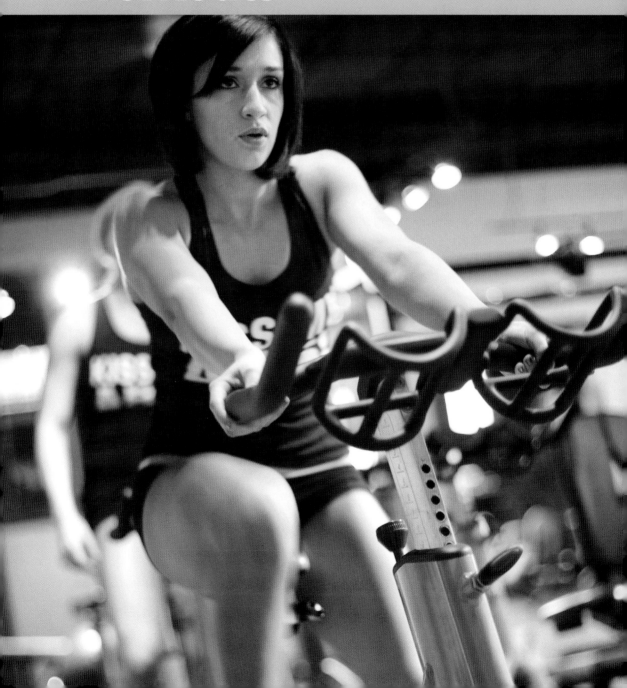

# Michael Friedman's View

Michael Friedman is a member of the Optum Pro Cycling Team presented by Kelly Benefits, U.S. National Champion in track racing, and an Olympian.

Many people loath the indoor trainer and refuse to spend any time using one. I used to be one of those people. Indoor trainers took up a lot of room. They were also loud (some still are), cumbersome to move about, and completely boring. Over the past 15 years of my riding career, the indoor trainer has changed considerably, and so has my mentality toward using them specifically as a training device. Today, I rarely get on the trainer to just ride without having a goal, and I'm never bored anymore.

I've traveled to over 32 countries racing and training, and I'm not always in an ideal place to train effectively. I've found that the trainer is a very useful tool, especially when I'm working on specifics such as climbing. Although it's probably one of my worst attributes as a cyclist, I was born with this body, and what goes up slower comes down faster. To drag myself over some of the courses I race on, I need to train specifically for climbing.

I live in Colorado now and have access to some of the best canyon riding available, but you might not have access to roads like the ones I'm used to. Or you may find yourself in this situation: The weather is poor, and your cycling coach says you need to do 4 × 15-minute climbing intervals, negative splitting the second half of the climb. This is where the trainer is effective.

On a trainer, the efforts are more controllable than when doing the effort on an actual climb. There is no wind, no traffic, no obstacles, and no fluctuations in power due to undulations in the gradient. You can work on cadence variations, accelerations, steady state, aerobic, anaerobic, climbing positions (in and out of the saddle), pedal stroke during efforts, and so on.

During your efforts, nobody is watching you. You can become a quitter on your own dime and stop the interval; or you can grow your mental fortitude, push through the effort, and finish the job. I say that because quitting is addictive—once you do it once, it's much easier the second and third time. I've found that I can work on that "never quit" attitude during many of my trainer sessions. A number of factors are at play on this. I typically find that the efforts on the trainer feel much harder than riding on the road. These efforts mentally crack me time after time.

Everyone has their own routine to help make riding in place more sustainable, whether it involves music, fans, TV, or the workout itself. I'm no different, but I try to keep the time limited. I don't do more than an hour and a half on the trainer, and I try to make it painful in order to make the time go by faster. When I get off the trainer, I will be dizzy and light-headed, knowing that I accomplished what I set out to do; only after doing the hard work indoors and out do I feel ready and confident when I'm on a starting line.

**Training** indoors provides many advantages. Weather, time constraints, and the desire to do certain types of workouts are all reasons for making indoor workouts a vital part of your training program. Even if you prefer to ride outside, you'll have to agree that sometimes the indoor trainer is the better option or even the necessary option.

While rollers help with your form and technique, fixed trainers (e.g., wind, resistance, or magnetic trainers) offer added stability that allows you to focus on other aspects of your ride besides keeping the bike upright. Many riders have strong preferences on the type of trainer they like to ride, so you should test out various options before making your purchase. Most trainers can change resistance on the fly. Using this control in addition to your standard bicycle gearing will allow you to complete the intervals included in this chapter.

One of the toughest things about riding a trainer is boredom (at least for me and my ADD mind). Sure, you can put on a DVD and race a stage of the Tour de France with your heroes, but on the days when you feel less enthusiastic, the workouts presented here will make the time fly by. Once you get a good foundation of workouts, you should try to come up with new and clever ways to make the workout interesting. Vary the workouts to fulfill your needs. I used to do my intervals to music. I'd forget about the clock and just go off the verse and chorus. Chorus was "game on," and the verse was rest. You don't even want to know what happened during the bridge!

Riding a trainer is mentally challenging. Outside, you deal with terrain, wind, and obstacles—all the things you expect on a bike ride. Inside, you deal with the dull hum of your wheel spinning, no air cooling (unless you hook up a fan), and the unrelenting resistance of your trainer. Maybe because riding inside feels artificial, some riders struggle to find motivation. But that's part of the training. Cycling has a huge mental component, and riding inside makes you a tougher bike rider. Just like getting caught in a rainstorm, getting up after a crash, or pushing yourself to the limit on a climb, riding inside on the trainer helps you become mentally tough.

If you live in a place where it snows or freezes, the trainer is invaluable for preventing lapses in your training. As described earlier, one of the components of the RACE philosophy is consistency. There's no point in losing out just because Mother Nature has made the weather unbearable. The tough part is that if you buy a trainer, you no longer have an excuse to go out for a hot chocolate instead of slipping on the biking shorts.

Another component of the RACE philosophy is efficiency—making the most of your time on the bike. The indoor trainer is a no-nonsense tool. It gets the job done straightaway. If you're feeling pressure from work or family, or if you can only work out after dark, the trainer becomes an invaluable option.

A lot of riders actually enjoy the trainer. They say it mixes things up and gives them a chance to focus on things that they forget about during outdoor rides. They can give their full attention to form or effort. Some ride in front of a mirror to see how they look when riding with their hands on various positions of the handlebar—tops, hoods, drops.

A big benefit of the indoor trainer is that it allows you to make quick changes in your workout. You don't have to worry about traffic, unfortunate timing of terrain, or momentum changes of the bike. One-leg riding is also totally feasible. In addition, you can make quick transitions for interval patterns, and you can hit the shower immediately after your cool-down.

Spinning classes have become a mainstay at every gym, and the instructors are fantastic at mixing things up. I went with my wife not too long ago and came home exhausted. That trainer kicked my butt! If you belong to a gym or club, you should check out the spin classes. You can take some of the workouts home and incorporate them into your own routine.

## Cycling Spotlight

Rollers are smooth, real smooth. They are a great way to ensure that you have a well-rounded pedal stroke. Any excess movement on the saddle or uneven pressure on the pedals becomes quickly apparent on the rollers. You have to pay attention when riding rollers. If you space out or get lost in a movie on the TV, you can ride straight off. Not only can you hurt yourself, but the bike will put a nasty hole in the drywall! (That too, I know from experience.)

A trainer is a bit easier to manage and certainly more stable. But just because you're locked in at the hub, that doesn't mean you can forget about your form. All of your trainer workouts offer you a perfect opportunity to look closely at your form. As mentioned earlier, some riders use a mirror to check out their position. This is not vanity; it's smart and functional. If you have your trainer in the bathroom and your roommate or significant other comes home wondering what's going on, you can just say, "Dr. Sovndal told me to do it."

| | |
|---|---|
| **Total Time** | 30 to 40 minutes |
| **Warm-Up** | 10 minutes |
| **Terrain** | Trainer |
| **Training Zone** | 5 |
| **Workout Time** | 10 to 20 minutes |
| **Cool-Down** | 10 minutes |

This is a rapidly changing interval. Each interval is done in zone 5. Start in the little chainring in the front. Your cadence should be greater than 115 to 120 rpm. After 15 seconds, switch to the big ring in the front. Your cadence will drop below 90 to 100. After 15 more seconds, switch back to the little ring; then, again after 15 seconds, go to the big ring. The total "on" time is 60 seconds. Take a break for 60 seconds, and then hit it again. This is a big advantage of the trainer. It allows you to make rapid transitions from high to low cadence. You shouldn't have to change the rear derailleur gearing. The only switch that needs to be made is the front chainring.

Chocolate milk is a great recovery food. Not only does it taste fantastic, but it has been shown to be as effective as some fancy recovery drinks. Chocolate milk contains protein, sugar, and some fat—all the ingredients that your body is craving.

STATIONARY BIKE

# TRULY SINGLE

Try to find riding partners who motivate you. Whether you're riding by yourself or with others, you can share your workouts and push each other to better and better performances. Websites are available that enable you to track your rides and your friends' rides. This way, everyone in the group of friends can see how far the others are progressing.

| | |
|---|---|
| **Total Time** | 32 to 36 minutes |
| **Warm-Up** | 10 minutes |
| **Terrain** | Trainer |
| **Training Zone** | 3 |
| **Workout Time** | 12 to 16 minutes |
| **Cool-Down** | 10 minutes |

Don't let your significant other panic when he or she hears you talking about Truly Single. Make it clear that this is just another crazy exercise to make you ride ever faster. In a previous workout, you did intervals on the road where you applied pressure with only one leg. Now you'll do it for real on the trainer. Unclip one leg and rest it on a chair next to the trainer. Make sure the crank doesn't strike your leg as it comes around. This is a slow-motion, muscle sensation workout. You should concentrate on the various muscles of your leg firing as the crank rotates through 360 degrees. Feel your quads, hamstrings, calf, and anterior lower-leg muscles each contribute. Notice the position of your foot as it rotates. Does your heel come up or stay down? Do this rotation only as fast as you can while still sensing the movement and keeping the correct form. Do 2 minutes and then switch sides. Do at least three or four intervals on each side. You can incorporate this into another trainer workout if you'd like.

| | |
|---|---|
| **Total Time** | 28 minutes |
| **Warm-Up** | 10 minutes |
| **Terrain** | Trainer |
| **Training Zone** | 2 |
| **Workout Time** | 8 minutes |
| **Cool-Down** | 10 minutes |

The point of this workout is similar to Truly Single. You are trying to gain a real sense of all the muscle groups spinning as you rotate your cranks. This is more of a form exercise than a true workout, but you should revisit it regularly. Spin in an easy gear for 30 to 60 seconds. Immediately switch to a reverse spin for 30 to 60 seconds. Freewheel backward. Repeat at least four times. Again, the point is to focus on the movement of your legs and the activation of your muscle groups. Be as smooth as possible, and only go as fast as good form will allow you.

Dizzy is an awesome exercise to incorporate into another workout. Add this workout onto the tail end of another easy workout and then do the same after a hard training exercise. Focus on the different sensations. You'll have a more difficult time being smooth after the hard workout because all your accessory muscles that help hold perfect form will be fatigued.

A nice way to work out is to set up your trainer in front of the TV and put on a video of a Tour de France stage. Work your intervals and training into the race. You'll feel as if you're racing with the pros—right there in your living room!

STATIONARY BIKE

Learn to recover while moving. After an effort, don't think that you need to completely stop in order to start your recovery. As you decrease your effort below your threshold, your body will start the recovery process. This is what happens when you watch a race and see the riders attack, sit in, and then attack again. Apply this active recovery to your exercise regime, and you'll be amazed at how much you can do and still recover.

| | |
|---|---|
| **Total Time** | 30 to 45 minutes |
| **Warm-Up** | 10 minutes |
| **Terrain** | Trainer |
| **Training Zone** | 6 |
| **Workout Time** | 15 to 30 minutes |
| **Cool-Down** | 5 minutes |

Remember your LT test? This is similar except you'll ramp up your speed every 30 seconds. Start at an easy speed—13 to 15 mph. Find a good cadence of 90 to 100 rpm. Start your timer. Every 30 seconds, increase your mph by 1. You may use your gears to obtain the required speed. The interval ends when you can't maintain the speed for the full 30 seconds. Yes, as you suspected, this is going to hurt. The duration will depend on your fitness and ability, but you should run through this interval at least two times. Rest fully (3 to 5 minutes) between intervals. If you can get three or even four intervals, then that's fantastic. This is an incredible test of your fitness level and is absolutely individualized. If you repeat this workout at regular intervals and track your performance in your diary, you will be stoked when you review your progress. You'll increase your speed and the duration of the interval training. Record your maximal speed for this interval. You'll use it in the next workout.

| | |
|---|---|
| **Total Time** | 30 minutes to 1 hour |
| **Warm-Up** | 10 minutes |
| **Terrain** | Trainer |
| **Training Zone** | 5 |
| **Workout Time** | 10 to 30 minutes |
| **Cool-Down** | 10 minutes |

Just when you thought things couldn't get worse, this workout requires you to ramp up your interval only to bring it back down. The first half is similar to Ramp Up. Once you reach your maximum speed, you'll slow your pace in the reverse order, slowing 1 mph every 30 seconds.

You don't have to go quite as fast as you did in the Ramp Up workout, but you will use your maximal speed from that workout as a reference point. Start your interval at an easy pace—15 or 16 mph. Every 30 seconds, increase your speed by 1 mph. You may use your gears to help you obtain your speed and desired cadence. Your maximum speed will be 2–4 mph less than your maximum speed during Ramp Up. Once you've ridden for 30 seconds at the maximal speed, decrease 1 mph every 30 seconds until you return to your starting point. Depending on your condition, you may only be able to do one "V" ramp up and down. If you can do more, then knock yourself out.

When you shift gears, let off a bit of the power. If you are going full tilt and driving the pedals hard, the derailleur may not be able to handle the pressure. Whether climbing or doing intervals, you should ease back for a moment when you make the switch and then get back on the gas. You can practice this on the road or trainer until you are able to perform it smoothly. Failed shifting can cost you a race—just ask Andy Schleck about the 2010 Tour de France.

STATIONARY BIKE

# TIME . . . OUT

Every day, you should do something to prove that you're tough. At some point during the day, force yourself to be better than expected. It can be a tiny thing or a big one. Just push yourself that extra inch. By doing this, you will know that when you are put to the test, you have a habit of proving to yourself that you are tough.

| | |
|---|---|
| **Total Time** | 30 to 45 minutes |
| **Warm-Up** | 15 minutes |
| **Terrain** | Trainer |
| **Training Zone** | 6 |
| **Workout Time** | 6 to 18 minutes |
| **Cool-Down** | 10 minutes |

This workout will give you progressively less and less rest while performing intervals. The idea is to teach your body to deal with the burn. All the waste products of hard exercise, along with accumulating muscle fatigue, will force you to adapt to physiologic conditions that are less than ideal.

After your warm-up, perform maximally for 30 seconds, then rest for 1 minute. Get back on the throttle for 30 seconds, but this time, rest for 45 seconds. Each time you rest, it will be shorter and shorter. Go full gas for 30 seconds, then rest for 30 seconds. Next, go full gas for 30 seconds, rest for 15 seconds, then perform a final 1-minute interval. When you've completed a whole cycle, rest for at least 5 minutes before repeating.

| | |
|---|---|
| **Total Time** | 30 to 45 minutes |
| **Warm-Up** | 15 minutes |
| **Terrain** | Trainer |
| **Training Zone** | 5 |
| **Workout Time** | 6 to 18 minutes |
| **Cool-Down** | 10 minutes |

This interval changes rapidly—20 seconds riding with full effort, followed by 20 seconds of recovery spin. You'll go back and forth, effort followed by recovery. Perform these intervals in groups of five (one set). That means you'll do five intervals of 20 seconds on, 20 seconds of recovery. After the five repetitions, take at least a 5-minute break to recover more fully. Depending on your fitness level, you should do between one and three sets.

This workout is a bit like a criterium race, where riders are accelerating out of corners, sitting in the pack for recovery, and then hitting the gas again. Even if you don't race, this interval works all your high-end energy systems. You'll become more fluid switching between hard and easy efforts, and your physiology will become adept at rapidly reenergizing after a hard effort.

No workout needs to be set in stone. As you progress through the various workouts in this book, you'll find what works for you and what doesn't. Keep notes in your training log and start coming up with new workouts that incorporate the best aspects as they apply specifically to you.

STATIONARY BIKE

# FRONT–BACKS

If possible, do some of your trainer riding in front of a mirror. You'll be able to really study your position on the bike without having to worry about crashing (although I have fallen off the rollers a few times, and it isn't pretty!).

| | |
|---|---|
| **Total Time** | 35 to 45 minutes |
| **Warm-Up** | 10 minutes |
| **Terrain** | Trainer |
| **Training Zone** | 4 |
| **Workout Time** | 11 to 22 minutes |
| **Cool-Down** | 10 minutes |

This interval is technical and a bit tedious, but it will help you improve your form. For 2 minutes, only pedal on the front half of the circle made by the revolution of your cranks—from 12 o'clock to 6 o'clock. Do this symmetrically with both legs at the same time. Now pedal for 2 minutes in complete circles (as described in chapter 14). Focus intently on your form. For the next 2-minute phase, you should pedal only the back half of the circle made by your crank rotation—from 6 o'clock to 12 o'clock. You'll be pulling up on the cranks only. You need to have clipless pedals or toe clips to perform this exercise. Finally, pedal in complete smooth circles for 5 minutes. Repeat the whole cycle if desired.

| | |
|---|---|
| **Total Time** | 30 to 45 minutes |
| **Warm-Up** | 15 minutes |
| **Terrain** | Slight incline on trainer |
| **Training Zone** | 5 |
| **Workout Time** | 6 to 18 minutes |
| **Cool-Down** | 10 minutes |

Raise the front wheel of your bike up off the ground 6 to 10 inches (15 to 25 cm) while it's attached to your trainer. (If you use rollers, you're out of luck with this one.) Increase the resistance so that you're working hard to maintain a cadence of 85 to 90 rpm. Climb for 10 minutes followed by 2 minutes of rest (decrease resistance and shift into an easy gear). Repeat if possible.

You are simulating climbing on your trainer. Like a lot of the trainer exercises, this workout focuses on your form. For the entire 10-minute interval, keep your hands on the tops of your handlebars. Slide back slightly in your saddle so you can really drive the cranks with some power. Focus on being smooth, and keep your shoulders from rocking or bouncing. If you really want to hone in your form, do this interval in front of a mirror so you can watch your form as you ride.

Don't think to yourself *I'm a climber* or *I'm a time trialist.* That closes down some of your potential. Many riders in the pro peloton started in one specialty but ultimately excelled in another. You should work on all aspects of your riding, especially when you are just getting serious about cycling.

STATIONARY BIKE

# Intervals

Keep in mind that you can mimic any of the other workouts while on a trainer. Pull any of the workouts from the previous chapters and apply them to the trainer. You'll find that a workout feels much different on a trainer than on the road. The trainer is mentally challenging, and the seconds seem to move slowly. It's amazing how much more you seem to sweat because you don't have the cooling effects of the wind.

You'll also be able to focus more on your form while riding a trainer because you don't have to worry about where you are going. As mentioned earlier, riding in front of a mirror is very helpful. Seeing the way you look on a bike, especially when doing a hard effort, will help you improve your form.

Riding on a trainer is a great time to try out new equipment. If something doesn't feel or fit just right, you don't have to suffer through it for an entire ride. Just hop off, fix the problem, and away you go on the trainer again.

## Sample Stationary Bike Program

| Week | Mon | Tues | Wed | Thurs | Fri | Sat | Sun |
|------|-----|------|-----|-------|-----|-----|-----|
| 1 | Off or gym | Time . . . Out Pg. 138 | Dizzy Pg. 135 | Off or gym | Climb to Oblivion Pg. 141 | Cross-training | Double Time Pg. 80 |
| 2 | Off or gym | Full Gas Pg. 76 | Front–Backs Pg. 140 | Off or gym | High-Speed Switchers Pg. 133 | Truly Single Pg. 134 | Cross-training |
| 3 | Off or gym | Time . . . Out Pg. 138 | V Is for Victory Pg. 137 | Off or gym | Minutemen Pg. 79 | Cross-training | Dizzy Pg. 135 |
| 4 | Off or gym | Minutemen Pg. 79 | Truly Single Pg. 134 | Off or gym | Climb to Oblivion Pg. 141 | Front–Backs Pg. 140 | Long Johns Pg. 83 |

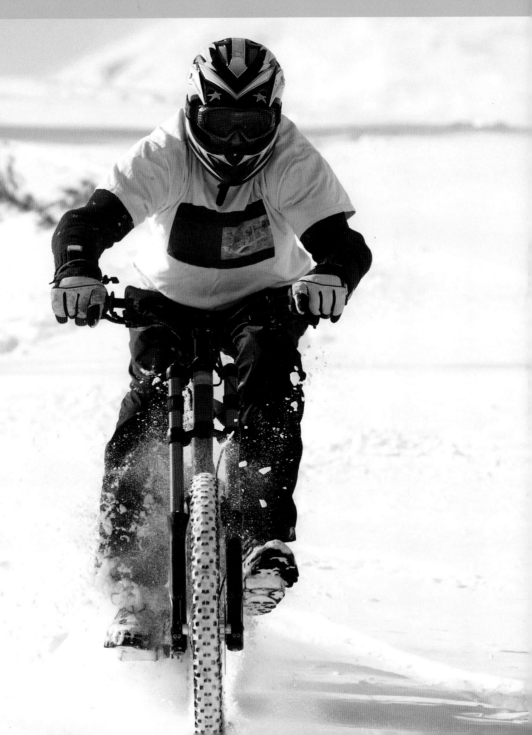

# Chris Baldwin's View

Chris Baldwin is a member of the Bissell Professional Cycling Team, a two-time U.S. national TT champion, and winner of the Tour of the Gila.

Ahhh, "off-season"—as far as bike racers are concerned, these are two of the greatest words ever spoken! Although most pros are passionate about the sport to the point of fanaticism, they all look forward to a break after a full campaign of racing and training. I would compare the feeling to getting out of school for summer break—that beautiful sensation of being able to let your guard down and do the things you put off all season. It's a time to let the focus go and recharge for the next round. For the guys I know, this time is commenced with a cheeseburger, a trip to a beach, or a night out on the town.

The off-season, or time off the bike, is different for everyone. Every cyclist has different needs, tastes, and obligations for this period.

Long ago, I was advised to take a full 4 weeks completely off from the bike. At first this sounded like a recipe for losing all my hard-earned fitness. But I took the advice and realized that the physical and mental break was like supercharging my batteries down the road. Not only that, but the fitness came back surprisingly quickly. I only changed this template once in my career, shortening my break to 2 weeks in an attempt to "get a head start" on the next season. It had the opposite effect. I started the year with more fatigue and low motivation. I have actually ADDED a week the last few years!

After a few weeks off, I hike a bit or maybe hit a yoga class. I certainly don't structure this time though. I can't lie, during this break I don't do much. I eat some junk food, catch up on house repairs, and have the beers I've been avoiding. My wife and I try to get away for some quality time without the bike. But by the end, I am ready to attack my training with vigor, eager to try to reach a new level the following season.

**Once** the season or macrocycle is complete, you need to assess and rejuvenate. You've spent a lot of time trying to reach your goals, and now is the time to sit back and look at the big picture. Did you reach your goals? Did you stick with the program? What were your strengths and weaknesses? What were some unforeseen limitations that hindered your progress?

All of these questions will help you better prepare your training program the next time around. Take a look through your training log and review all that you've accomplished. In your training journal, list three things that worked and then three things that you need to change for next season. Write them down while things are still fresh. You don't want to forget something that will contribute to your success in the years to come.

# Phase 1: Vacation

The off-season should be broken into two phases. The first is referred to as a vacation from the bike. Let your mind and body recover from all the days you've spent training and riding. You'll feel better and more focused when you come back to start your new season. Even if you're gung ho and can't wait for the next season to start, force yourself to step away from cycling.

During this phase, you should put away everything related to cycling. After your initial evaluation of the previous training year, put the training journal away. Hang up the bike and close up the mechanics bench. You need a few weeks to clear your mind and focus on something other than riding your bike. Let go of any shortcomings during the previous training year, and enjoy not having a training schedule. The vacation can last 2 to 4 weeks. Keep in mind that you can stay active; it just shouldn't be on the bike. You shouldn't have any sort of structure to your activities. Let your mind chill and just relax . . . chillax.

# Phase 2: Base Fitness and Strength Training

After you've had your vacation, it is time to start the second phase of the off-season and work to maintain a baseline level of fitness. This phase can also last 2 to 4 weeks. It will vary a bit based on the length of your vacation. You should be aiming to take a 4- to 8-week break from serious riding during the off-season. Choose any activity that strikes your fancy. Conditioning in the off-season should be fun, entertaining, and refreshing. The only requirement here is that you need to do exercises other than cycling. It's perfectly fine to go out on a ride now and again, but the bulk of your cardio work should be performed in activities without a bike.

Training consistently in one sport during the course of the season will cause certain muscles and systems to develop. During the off-season, you should work to build and strengthen some of the muscles that cycling neglects. Choose activities that will provide a base of cardiovascular fitness that you can build on once you start to train. Run, hike, swim, cross-country ski, snowshoe—do anything that will keep your heart rate elevated.

These workouts do not have to be regimented, but each week you should try to get in at least two or three workouts of 30 to 60 minutes. Again, the specific activity isn't important. Just do anything that makes your aerobic system do some work. Some activities, such as downhill skiing or pickup basketball, won't even seem like a workout. You'll be having too much fun!

## Core Strength

During the second phase of the off-season, you should also start focusing on gym work. This is the perfect time to increase your core strength and cycling power. Start your workouts by building core power. This can be done by going to workout classes at a local gym, doing yoga or Pilates, meeting with a personal trainer, or just going to the gym. The focus shouldn't be on lifting heavy weights, but rather on gaining core strength and flexibility.

Try to work out two or three times a week, always taking a break between workouts. During the off-season, you can combine core workouts with base fitness training.

Core fitness will prevent injury and overuse issues during the season; it will also enable you to leap into your training from a higher baseline. If you have the time, you should incorporate activities such as yoga or Pilates. Both strengthen your foundation and allow for more training load in the future.

The following section provides some sample exercises that focus on building a strong core. A stability ball or balance disc is very useful in core workouts. If you don't have access to these at home or the gym, you can do most of the exercises directly on the floor. You'll likely have to do the medicine ball throw at a gym. Again, these workouts are just to give you an example. Feel free to talk to your friends or have a personal trainer direct you. The key is to work on your core muscles.

If you'd like further description and more individual weight training exercises, refer to my book *Cycling Anatomy* (Human Kinetics, 2009). It is full of specific training exercises based on each muscle group. It also helps you understand each exercise's applicability to your cycling performance.

# Sample Core Exercises

## STABILITY BALL EXTENSION

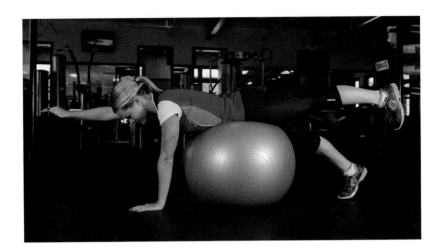

### Execution

1. Lie with your lower abdomen draped over a stability ball.
2. Keeping one foot on the floor, arch your back while raising and extending your arm and opposite leg. Your elbow and knee should be straight (extended).
3. Slowly lower your arm and leg. Curl your body around the stability ball.
4. Repeat the exercise using your other arm and leg.

### Exercise Notes

Your back extender muscles must withstand enduring workloads when you ride your bike. For the majority of your ride, these muscles will maintain your forward leaning posture. If your back becomes sore or fatigued, the back extender muscles are usually the culprit. The stability ball extension is particularly effective because it gives you full range of motion at maximal extension. This will counter the hours you'll spend with your back arched forward on the bike. Don't think that you need to use added weights to make this workout effective. Remember that stretching and moving your muscles through their complete range of motion will help you get the most out of your muscle fibers.

### Variation

**Same-side stability ball extension:** A good variation is to raise the arm and leg on the same side rather than on opposite sides as described for the main exercise. This will stress different stabilizers and give you a well-rounded workout.

## REVERSE LEG EXTENSION

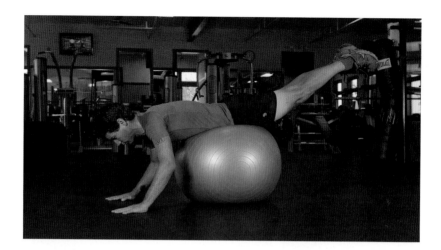

### Execution

1. Lie with your lower abdomen on a stability ball. Extend both arms forward, and place your palms on the floor. Your legs should be straight, and your toes should be resting on the floor.
2. Keeping your knees straight, slowly extend at the hip, elevating your legs off the ground.
3. Return to the starting position.

### Exercise Notes

As previously mentioned, cycling is tough on your lower back. In the gym, you should focus on developing these back muscles in order to avoid future aggravation. The stability ball is an excellent tool because it allows freedom of motion with the added benefit of working all the stabilizer muscles. Remember, a balanced musculature is the key to proper alignment and injury prevention. Because you are so confined in position during your time on the bike, you should perform more range-of-motion exercises in the gym. You'll ride faster and better if your body is balanced and your muscles have strength through their entire spectrum of movement.

## Variation

**Incline lumbar extension**: After you've been working this exercise for a while, you can hold weights to increase the difficulty. This exercise can also be done using an incline lumbar extension machine or bench. With the added stability, the workout for the stabilizer muscles is reduced.

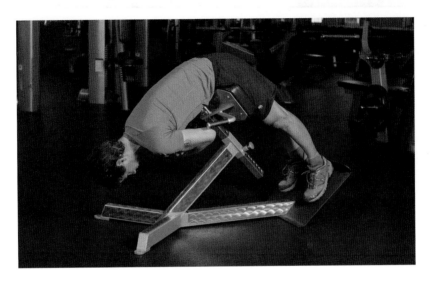

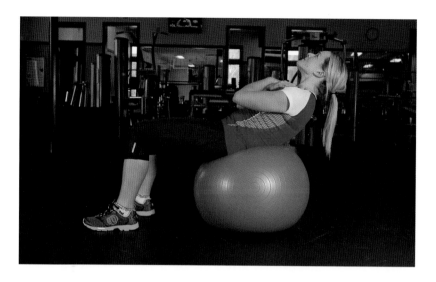

## Execution

1. Place your arms across your chest and rest your lower back on top of a stability ball. Your back and thighs should be horizontal and parallel with the floor. Your knees should be bent at 90 degrees, and your feet should be flat on the floor.
2. Lift your chin and torso upward as far as possible. Concentrate on moving your chin in a straight line toward the ceiling.
3. Pause briefly at your maximal height and then slowly return to the starting position.
4. For added difficulty, you can hold a medicine ball or weight plate with your arms outstretched over your chest throughout the entire motion.

## Exercise Notes

To deliver sustained power when riding your bike on a climb, you need to have a strong core that can handle the torque of your legs as they rotate through your pedal stroke. If you're delivering optimal power, you'll be pulling up with one leg while simultaneously crashing down with the other. At the same time, your arms will be pulling back and forth on the handlebars. Your core is the platform between your two sides, and the alternating movement of your legs and arms will naturally work to flex and destabilize your trunk. By maintaining a strong abdomen, you will help ensure that your upper body and pelvis can effectively fight against unnecessary movement. Any unwanted movement of your body or bike will lead to power loss and inefficiency. Even the best professionals only operate at near 27 percent efficiency, so saving your energy wherever possible is critical.

## Safety Tip

Keep your chin pointed upward toward the ceiling. Curling your chin down toward your chest will put undue strain on your cervical spine.

## Variation

**Side-to-side trunk lift**: Perform the same exercise, but instead of merely moving up and down, alternate lifting your body from side to side. This will not only work your primary abdominal muscles but will also focus on your stabilizer and lateral muscles. Again, to increase the difficulty of the exercise, you can hold a medicine ball or weight with outstretched arms above your chest as you lift your trunk.

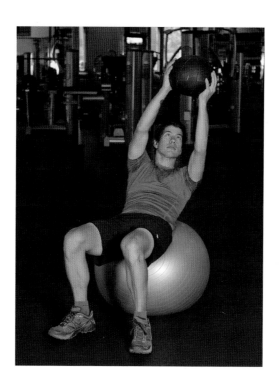

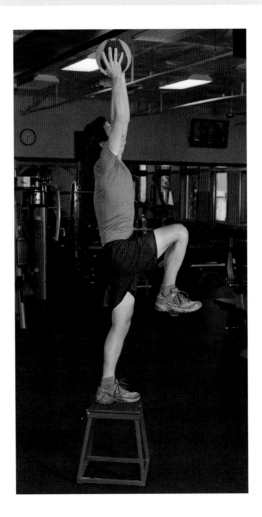

## Execution

1. Holding a medicine ball at your chest, stand in front of a platform.

2. With a forceful movement, step onto the platform. Drive your non-weight-bearing knee upward while extending your support leg. Simultaneously extend both your arms above your head. When finished, you should be standing on your tiptoes (on one leg) and holding the medicine ball over your head.

3. With controlled movement, step backward off the platform and return to your starting position.

4. Alternate your step-up leg.

## Exercise Notes

This exercise trains you to maintain your form while putting in a hard effort. When you step up and thrust the medicine ball above your head, all your stabilizer muscles fire. Because you're standing on only one leg while holding a load over your head, your pelvis must lock into position. This is similar to putting in a hard effort while riding. Whether you're seated or standing on the bike, your pelvis must provide a solid foundation to counteract the different actions of each of your legs. Because goalies involve the added effort of your torso and upper extremities, you'll also be training for the many hours of supporting your body weight over the handlebars.

## Variation

**Stairs and press:** If you have access to stairs in an arena or stadium, this is an excellent alternative to goalies. Hold a dumbbell in each hand. Skip every other step as you ascend the stairs. While climbing, perform an arm press with each dumbbell above your head. You can do this with both arms together or arms alternating.

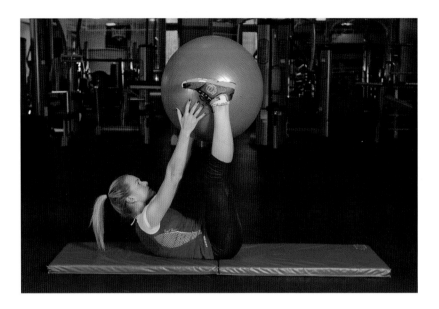

### Execution

1. Lie on your back with your legs extended. Squeeze a stability ball between your feet, and extend your arms horizontally above your head.
2. Perform a crunch motion, pulling your legs and arms to the vertical position. Your shoulders should come vertically off the floor.
3. Transfer the ball from your feet to your hands.
4. Slowly lower the ball in your hands to the starting position until your arms and legs are extended horizontally. Repeat.

### Exercise Notes

The importance of pelvis stability when riding a bike cannot be overemphasized. Whether you're sprinting, climbing, or time trialing, your legs rely on a strong foundation to enable them to generate their impressive force while rotating the cranks. During a time trial, your body should be still and solid as you slice through the wind in your aerodynamic position. The more power you can deliver to the pedals, the faster you'll ride. Your abdominal muscles will play a key role in establishing this needed base. The stability ball pass has the advantage of working some of your hip and leg muscles as well as your abdomen. By pushing your feet together to hold the ball, you will work your hip adductors. Good strength in both your adductors and abductors will help smooth your pedal stroke when you're fatigued or working at maximum capacity.

## MEDICINE BALL THROW

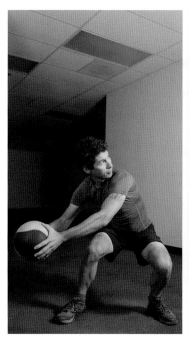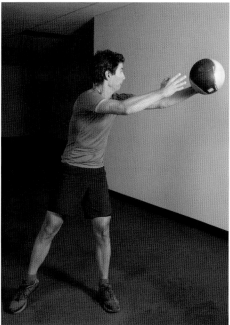

### Execution

1. Hold a medicine ball in both hands, and stand about 8 to 10 feet (2.4 to 3.0 m) in front of a wall.
2. Twist your trunk, crunch, and bring the ball back to one side. You should stand with one foot slightly ahead of the other.
3. With an explosive movement, extend and heave the ball at the wall.
4. Catch the ball after it bounces off the wall and rapidly repeat the action on the opposite side. Continue alternating until you finish the set.

### Exercise Notes

Cycling is all about surges. A surge at the right time can create a gap that may give you the opportunity to win the race. Imagine being on your bike and climbing with your competitors. You decide the time is now, and you make an explosive jump. After your acceleration, you're able to hold the speed for two minutes. Slowly, you back off and return to your previous pace. Although you may be climbing at the same speed as your competitors, you've got yourself a significant gap. Now you can try to hold it to the finish. The medicine ball throw will help you develop the explosive surge needed in order to make this kind of successful race move. Focus on the explosive nature of the throw. The word *heave* accurately describes what you need to do in this exercise. Throw that ball with all your might!

### Variation

**Squat with front throw:** Start in a squat position square to the wall while you hold a medicine ball at your chest. Surge to the standing position. At the same time, throw the ball at the wall in front of you. (Use a pushing motion on the ball, as if you're making a basketball pass.) Return to the starting position and repeat the action in rapid succession. To mix it up even further, you can perform the same exercise but throw the medicine ball forward from behind your head. The motion is similar to throwing a soccer ball over your head.

## Lifting for Cycling Power

After you've completed a few weeks of the core workouts, it's time to start working on your cycling-specific power. Your off-season goal should be to build raw power that you can transfer into cycling-specific speed and power on the bike. These are weight training exercises that will allow you to generate maximal power with each turn of the pedal stroke.

In-depth explanations of weight training are beyond the scope of this book, but some examples of key exercises for cyclists are provided in the following section. You should consider meeting with a personal trainer who can give you a complete program and ensure that you're doing the exercises correctly. Always start with low weights and work your way up. Whenever you work out in the gym, there is a potential risk of injury, so make sure you take your time building up the weight. Always sacrifice weight in order to maintain good form. If you can't do the exercise properly, it is better to hold off rather than injure yourself.

To build strength in the off-season, you should shoot for three weight training workouts per week. During each workout, do two or three sets of each exercise. Think of your weight training as being broken up into three separate strength phases. Books that focus entirely on weight training will present more complicated schemes, but this model works well if you are just getting started.

1. **Transitional phase.** This phase helps your ligaments, joints, and muscles adapt to the demands of weight training. You start out with light weights and allow time for your body to settle into gym work. This will be your first training phase, and it will also occur between blocks of the building phase. The initial phase will be 2 to 3 weeks; when a transitional phase is used between blocks of the building phase, the transitional phase will be 1 to 2 weeks.

2. **Building phase.** The building phase is when you'll really be doing some work. By performing fewer repetitions with heavier weights, you will build the strength that makes you ride better and faster. This phase lasts for 2 weeks. After the building phase, you'll go back to the transition phase for 1-2 weeks, before, once again, hitting a building phase.

3. **Maintenance phase.** This is the phase of strength training that occurs during most of the cycling season. After you've had multiple phases of transition and building, you'll be ready to spend more time on the bike. The regular training year will start, and you'll need to maintain the muscle strength that you've developed. The point of this phase is to maintain your current level as much as possible during the months when the focus of your training is not on gym work.

During the off-season, you'll bounce back and forth between numerous cycles of transition and building. The number of cycles will be dictated by your overall training plan and the amount of time you've dedicated to the gym. As a good starting point, you can plan to spend about 2 to 3 months in the gym before you start to spend considerably more time performing cycling-specific training (see table 12.1).

**Table 12.1   Strength Training Phases**

| Transition phase | Building phase | Maintenance phase |
|---|---|---|
| 2-3 weeks for initial phase | 2 weeks | All season |
| 15-20 repetitions | 6-10 repetitions | 10-12 repetitions |
| 3 sets | 2-3 sets | 2-3 sets |

# Sample Lifting Exercises

## MACHINE LEG PRESS

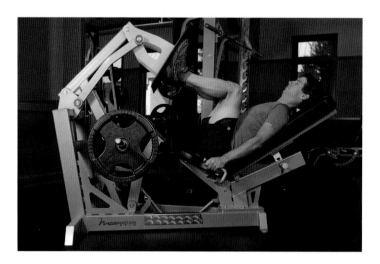

### Execution

1. Sit on the sled with your feet shoulder-width apart and your back flat against the padded seat.
2. Slowly bend your knees and lower the weight until your knees are at a 90-degree angle.
3. Extend your legs and return the weight to its original position. (Don't lock your knees.)

### Exercise Notes

This is a cyclist's bread-and-butter leg exercise. The leg press machine allows you to work on your upward surge and helps develop explosive cycling power. The solid back support helps prevent injury when accelerating out of your squat position. Change your foot position to emphasize different muscles of your lower extremity. Place your feet high on the footplate to train your gluteus maximus and hamstrings. A low foot position emphasizes your quadriceps. Adjust stance width to train various muscles. A wide stance especially works your inner quad, and accessory hip muscles including your hip adductors. A narrow stance puts the focus on your outer quad and hip abductors.

### Variation

**Hack squat:** While standing, position your back flat against the sliding back rest. Wedge your shoulders snugly under the pads. Slowly perform a squat. The hack squat places added emphasis on your quadriceps. Like the leg press, you can switch between squats, calf extensions, and reverse calf raises. You can also exercise one leg at a time to ensure equal training.

## SPLIT-LEG SQUAT

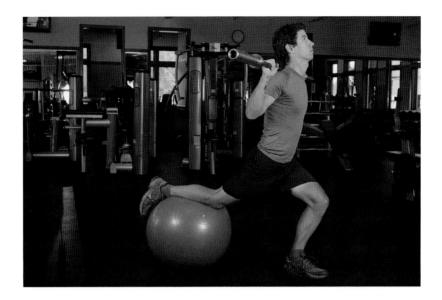

### Execution

1. While standing, place a barbell over your shoulders.
2. Place one foot slightly forward. Extend your other leg back, placing it on top of a stability ball.
3. Slowly bend your front knee until it makes a 90-degree angle. Return to the standing position.

### Exercise Notes

Imagine climbing up a steep grade and having to accelerate to match an attack from another rider. You'll need to maximize your entire pedal stroke to meet the challenge. Split-leg squats will help you develop powerful quadriceps, which will enable you to deliver a strong kick over the top of your pedal stroke. This is also an important exercise for cyclists because it lets them train each leg individually. Without knowing it, cyclists often have one leg that is disproportionately stronger than the other. This can be hidden when the cyclist is performing exercises that use both legs simultaneously. In the split-leg squat, any inequalities will be recognized and can be remedied through training.

### Variations

**Split-leg squat with bench:** For more stability, you can place your rear foot on a bench. This will help if you are finding it difficult to keep your balance while doing the exercise with a stability ball.

**Smith machine split-leg squat:** The Smith machine is another more stable option. Using the Smith machine will help stabilize your movement. It will also help protect your back and provide you with an artificial spotter.

## LEG EXTENSION

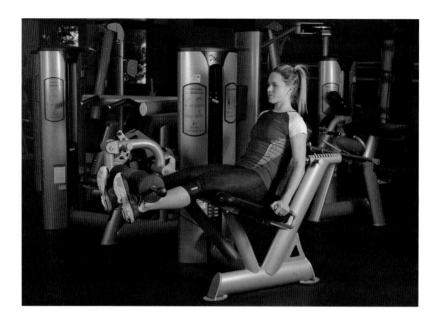

### Execution

1. Sit on the machine with the middle of your knee aligned with the pivot point.
2. Raise your legs until your knees are straight. Your toes should be pointed upward.
3. After a brief pause, return to the starting position (knees bent to 90 degrees).

### Exercise Notes

The next time you go out on a ride, try to feel your various leg muscles firing while you are pedaling at a steady rate. Try to do the same during a fierce acceleration in a sprint or a climb. You'll note that as your leg kicks over the top of the pedal stroke, your quadriceps will fire with a vengeance. You'll also be able to feel the similarity between this part of your pedaling motion and the motion used on the leg extension machine. This exercise isolates one of your major cycling muscles. Look at the development of any serious rider's quads, and you'll realize just how much these muscles are used during riding.

### Safety Tip

To avoid lower back injury, keep your spine flat against the machine pad.

## LYING LEG CURL

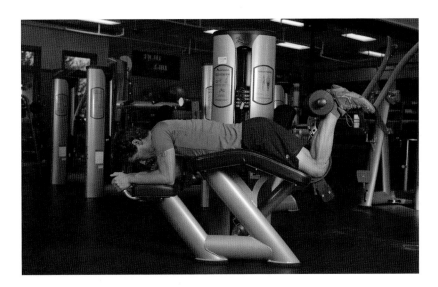

### Execution

1. Lay on the machine so the middle of your knee is aligned with the pivot point.
2. Keeping your stomach and pelvis flat on the pad, flex at the knees until they are bent past 90 degrees.
3. After a brief pause, return to the starting position (knees straight).

### Exercise Notes

The efficiency of the pedal stroke requires the constantly alternating and combined effort of both your legs. As one leg is emphasizing pulling, the other is emphasizing pushing. Just as the leg extension exercise replicates the top and front part of your pedal stroke, the leg curl focuses on the bottom and back part of your pedaling motion. As you lay on the leg curl machine, imagine pulling your foot through the bottom arc of your pedal stroke. Feel the similarity between the exercise motion and the upward pull you perform when completing a revolution of the crank. Be sure you don't "cheat" on this exercise by arching your back or pulling your pelvis off the pad into the air. Remember, the purpose is to isolate the hamstrings and give them the best training possible.

### Variation

**Seated leg curl:** The seated leg curl also is good at isolating your hamstrings. Feel free to use whichever machine is available at your gym.

## WALL STABILITY BALL SQUAT

### Execution

1. While standing, place the stability ball between your lower back and the wall.
2. Hold two dumbbells in your hands with your arms straight at your sides.
3. Perform a squat motion, bending your knees to 90 degrees. The ball will roll as you squat.
4. Return to the starting position.

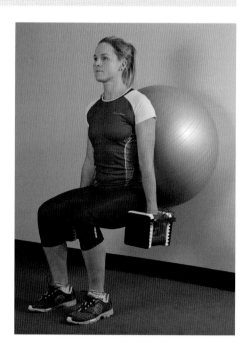

### Exercise Notes

This exercise not only helps you develop strong pistons to drive the pedals, but also emphasizes your abdominal muscles, back muscles, and lower extremity stabilizers. Because the stability ball can roll any direction on the wall, you'll be forced to control your foundation as you lift the weight. This instability helps strengthen your core and prepares you for the later miles of your rides. When you become tired, your form can start to fail, and your efficiency will drop. The longer you can prevent this from occurring, the better results you'll have.

### Variations

**Timed squat:** Position yourself as described, but don't use the dumbbells. Rather than do repetitions, proceed to the down position and hold it for a fixed amount of time. For example, you could hold the position for 30 seconds, 1 minute, 2 minutes, or more depending on your strength and conditioning.

**Squat on stability discs:** For some real instability, perform the timed exercise while standing on two stability discs. This places even greater emphasis on all your accessory muscles.

## Sample Off-Season Program

| Week | Mon | Tues | Wed | Thurs | Fri | Sat | Sun |
|------|-----|------|-----|-------|-----|-----|-----|
| 1 | Gym | Cross-training | Gym | Free | Gym | Cross-training | Free |
| 2 | Gym | Free | Gym | Cross-training | Gym | Free | Cross-training |
| 3 | Gym | Cross-training | Gym | Free | Gym | Cross-training | Free |
| 4 | Gym | Free | Gym | Cross-training | Gym | Free | Cross-training |

For more exercises and variation, check out my book *Cycling Anatomy* (Human Kinetics, 2009). It breaks up exercises by various muscle groups and helps guide you if you want more complete and varied workouts.

# Equipping Yourself

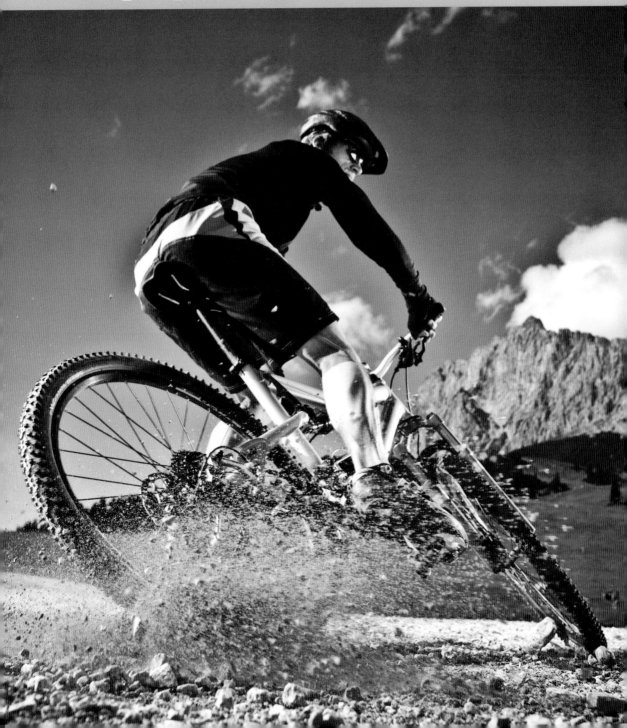

**So** many roads and trails to ride, but so little time. As mentioned earlier, this book is all about the performance rider. The goal is to help you get the most out of every ride. That all starts at the foundation: equipment.

You will need to outfit yourself for comfort, performance, and the type of riding you want to focus on. Equipment options are abundant, and if you're just getting started, they can seem a bit overwhelming. This chapter gives you some sound advice and information on the various types of equipment that will help you thoroughly enjoy your rides. Familiarize yourself with the various parts and components of the bike before you shop (figure 13.1). This will help you better evaluate the best bike model for you.

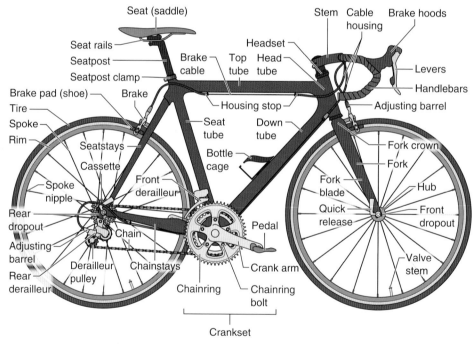

**Figure 13.1**  Parts of the bike.

# Choosing the Right Bike

The bicycle, and specifically the frame, is the foundation of all your equipment. Obviously, this is the most important purchase you'll make. So if you're on a tight budget, spend the majority of your funds on getting a high-quality bike. Upgrades, accessories, and add-ons will always be available at a later time.

Your first major decision is the type of bike that will best suit the majority of your riding. Road bikes are sleek, fast, and efficient. Their purpose is riding on paved roads. They are light, stiff, and comfortable. Whether you're climbing, descending, or just pumping away on the flats, road bikes are designed for speed.

Mountain bikes are specifically engineered for trails, dirt, and off-road riding. They are rugged, controllable, and shock absorbent. Even if you know you want a mountain bike, the decision is still complicated. Many options are available, including hardtails, dual suspensions, and 29ers. Each offers specific advantages that will be discussed in this chapter.

Time trialing (TT) has gained popularity over the past few years, in large part because of triathlons. TT bikes are highly specialized for aerodynamic efficiency. If your focus is riding solo at maximal effort, then the TT bike will give you the best performance.

Cyclocross bikes are a combination of a road bike and a mountain bike. They are designed for riding in less-than-ideal conditions, and they are also light enough to pick up and carry. Some competitions that involve these bikes incorporate both riding and carrying the bike.

Touring bikes and hybrids are specifically designed for comfort and carrying loads—tents, packs, groceries, and briefcases. They are good for commuters, townies, and long-distance travelers.

Whichever style of bike you decide on, your next major decision will be the composition of the frame (see the sidebar). Technology has enhanced the types of metals and composites that make up frames, and each has specific characteristics. Steel, aluminum, carbon, and titanium are the most common, but there are a whole slew of others. I have even had the unique experience of riding on a bamboo frame.

Some manufacturers mix the various components on different parts of the frame. This can complicate your choice. Be sure to research the options on the Internet, ask around, and finally take a good test ride. Every rider is different, and what feels fantastic to one might not do it for another. Trust your own feelings while test riding. Nobody knows you better than you!

# Frame Material

Frame technology is amazing. In the past, bikes were made from steel. Now technology has allowed bike makers to expand to various metals and composites, all in the hope of decreasing weight and improving performance. In addition to being light, the best bike offers a comfortable ride, absorbing bumps on the road or trail, while never sacrificing stiffness for climbing, sprinting, and cornering. Here's how the various metals and composites measure up:

- **Steel**—Modern steel is strong, but with true stiffness comes extra weight. It offers a comfortable ride, damping vibrations and road bumps. New "air-hardened" steel decreases weight and improves stiffness. Tubes can easily be rewelded if something breaks, and small dents don't notably compromise stiffness. Steel does fatigue; the metal loses some of its strength over time.
  - **Pros**—Strong, comfortable, most affordable, easily repaired, classic
  - **Cons**—Heavy, fatigable, not ideal for heavy riders or sprinters, rust prone if the paint chips
- **Aluminum**—Aluminum is a very light yet still affordable metal. To compensate for aluminum's low density, bike tubes are usually thicker when compared with classic steel tubes. Much of the strength is engineered in the shape of the tube. The downside is that a dent can greatly reduce the strength and stiffness of the frame.
  - **Pros**—Light, affordable, easily shaped into aero forms, stiffness (even for bigger riders)
  - **Cons**—Rough ride, more fragile, difficult to repair, fatigable
- **Titanium**—Titanium has excellent properties for frame building. It is light, durable, and corrosive resistant; and it offers a comfortable ride. Many "titanium" bikes are actually a combination of titanium, aluminum, and vanadium.
  - **Pros**—Light, resilient, comfortable ride, no rust (so no paint needed)
  - **Cons**—Expensive, less stiff than aluminum and carbon fiber, difficult to repair
- **Carbon fiber**—Individual fibers are aligned in specific patterns and then glued together to give a carbon fiber tube its strength. Unlike metals in which strength is nearly the same in all directions, carbon fiber can be oriented to provide strength where needed. Engineers "wrap" the fiber according to the stresses placed on the bike by road and rider.
  - **Pros**—Easily moldable, strong, light, fatigue resistant, comfortable ride
  - **Cons**—Expensive, breakable, uncomfortable if made incorrectly

## Road Bikes

These are the bikes you see racing in the Tour de France. They are designed for smooth paved roads, and their main purpose is to help you get the most speed out of your pedal stroke. The position of the rider minimizes wind resistance and maximizes power output. If you plan on racing or riding to get the best time, the road bike is the bike for you.

Road bikes have skinny tires, narrow saddles, front and rear chainrings, and standard downward bending handlebars (figure 13.2). They are light and aerodynamic. Each component is designed to maximize efficiency while at the same time being comfortable enough for long rides.

Tire sizing can be confusing. Most road bikes have 700 millimeter, or 700c, diameter wheels (measured from the hub to the outside of the wheel along a spoke). The c is not an actual unit of measurement, but it comes from an old-school notation on French tires. Some other size variations, such as 650 millimeter and 27 inch, are available; however, my recommendation is to go with a 700c wheel. Some racing organizations mandate that the wheel be this size if you want to compete.

The second component of the wheel size is the tire width. Most racing bikes range from 18 to 32 millimeters. This is the widest distance of the tire measured side to side (perpendicular to the axis of rotation). You'll see this nomenclature when you buy tires or tubes: 700c × 18 mm or 700c × 28 mm. If you're wondering about the size of a tire on a bike, you can read the tire sidewall for the designation.

Road bikes have a wide range of gearing. This allows for optimal performance over varied road terrain. On a typical ride, you'll be equipped to

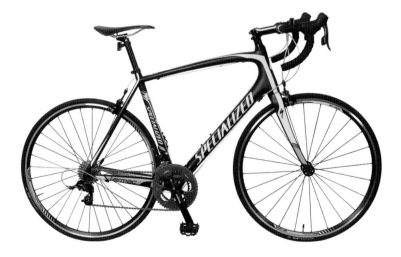

**Figure 13.2**   Road bike.

climb, descend at high speed, or cruise on the flats. If you compete, you'll also have the correct setup for sprinting.

Gearing ratios denote the combination of the front chainring and the rear chainring. (This is addressed further in the Gearing and Cadence section of chapter 14.) Road bikes have either two or three chainrings in the front; most racing bikes have only two. The rear hub commonly has 10-11 cogs.

Over the years, technology has allowed more and more cogs to efficiently fit on the hub. In the future, bikes will likely offer even more gearing options. The high number of gears may seem like overkill until you get out on the road and start riding over varied terrain. Using your gears appropriately will increase your efficiency and riding speed.

Saddles are extremely important. It might seem counterintuitive that road bikes have such narrow saddles, but for longer rides, the narrow saddle is more comfortable and efficient. You'll have more freedom of motion of your legs and less chafing on your inner thighs. With any of the bikes mentioned in this chapter, if you ride regularly, a narrow saddle is going to be your best option.

Keep in mind the importance of the saddle. You must ensure that it fits you well. You should consult your local bike shop or fellow riders for various options and best sellers. Based on their information, you can try out different setups to see which one best suits your anatomy. Here's a good tip: Never skimp on comfort to save weight. An uncomfortable saddle will certainly hinder your performance more than a few grams of extra weight.

## Mountain Bikes

Rough, off-road terrain is the playground of mountain bikes. They are tough, abuse-ready machines that absorb bumps, jumps, and unforgiving conditions. These bikes have geometries that favor stability and shock absorption, and they have wider tires to absorb and grip the terrain. Most models have some sort of suspension system—front, rear, or both. Because they are used on extreme terrain, most mountain bikes have a triple chainring in the front and 9 or 10 speeds in the rear.

Mountain bikes are now specialized. You can buy a downhill, cross-country, all-mountain, or free ride bike. Downhill mountain bikes are designed for speed and shock absorption when flying down a mountain. Cross-country bikes are the lightest and most efficient to pedal, but they may not offer the most comfort in truly rugged conditions. All-mountain bikes are designed as a compromise that will take you anywhere. They function well in most situations that you'll encounter on the trails. Free ride bikes are for stunts and terrain parks; they are for riders who specialize in big air and tricks. They aren't the most comfortable, and they are probably the most limited of the various types. My recommendation is to purchase a cross-country or all-mountain bike. These will serve you best for the widest range of terrain.

Modern mountain bikes usually come with some sort of suspension system. A hardtail has only a front shock incorporated into the fork. Different front shocks offer different amounts of "travel"—that is, the distance the shock moves up and down along the piston. Downhill bikes have more travel than cross-country or all-terrain bikes. A dual-suspension bike has a shock for the front fork and a shock system in the rear triangle (the triangle made by the seat tube, chainstays, and seat stays). Both hardtail and dual-suspension options have their advantages. Generally, hardtails climb better and are lighter, whereas dual-suspension bikes offer increased descent speed and a more comfortable ride.

To complicate matters further, you'll also need to decide between 26-inch wheels and 29-inch wheels. The original default size for mountain bikes was 26, but now 29ers are becoming extremely popular (figure 13.3).

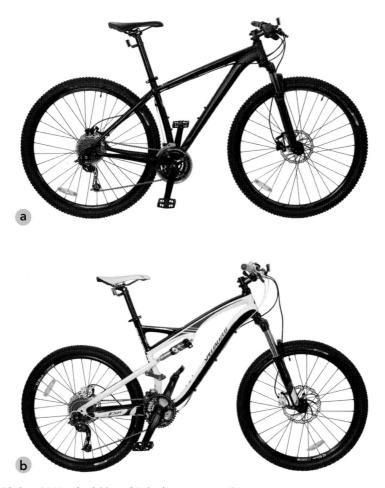

**Figure 13.3**    *(a)* Hardtail 29er; *(b)* dual-suspension 26.

There are pros and cons for each wheel size, and you can spend hours reading differing opinions on the Internet. A larger diameter tire can offer a smoother ride over rough terrain, but the 26-inch wheel makes the bike feel more nimble.

As with all sports, the more you ride, the more you'll be able to make a judgment about which type of bike suits your riding style. You just need to go ride the various models and see which one feels the best. Many avid cyclists have a "quiver" of bikes—hardtail, dual suspension, and various wheel sizes. In reality, you probably can't go wrong with any of them. The key is the test ride. Take it out and see how it feels. Get advice from various shops, friends, and online articles. Then, make your choice. If you love cycling, this probably won't be the last bike you ever purchase, so don't lose sleep at night trying to figure it out!

Mountain bike tires are wide and grippy. The tread pattern you select should depend on the type of terrain you'll spend most of your time riding on. Wide, very knobby treads work best for loose dirt and general mountain biking; tightly bunched square knobbies work best for extremely rocky terrain. Standard widths range from 1.8 to 2.5 inches (but you can find more extreme measurements on either end of the spectrum). Mountain bike tubes come in size ranges. If you check out a tube box in a store, you'll note something like this: 26 × 2.1-2.5. These tubes fit any tire labeled with a size that falls within that range. As with road bikes, you can find the size of the tire by looking at the numbers on the sidewall.

As mentioned, mountain bikes have a wide range of gears for handling the varied mountain terrain. A triple chainring in the front, coupled with 9 or 10 cogs in the rear, provides up to 30 different gears. In the past few years, it has become trendy in some areas to ride single-speed mountain bikes. These bikes have no shifting options. Although these single-speed bikes can be fun, a geared mountain bike is a much better option if you're just getting started.

## Time-Trialing Bikes

Racing solo against the clock requires maximal speed, aerodynamics, and efficiency. Time-trialing (TT) bikes are not the most versatile or comfortable, but they do their specific task well. The first time trial bikes were modified road bikes, but now you have a wide selection from various manufacturers of true time-trialing machines. They place the rider in a forward tucked position using a steep seat tube angle and aerobars (figure 13.4). The ride is stiff, enhancing the rider's ability to transfer all the energy to the drivetrain.

Like road bikes, TT bikes have 700c wheels. However, wheels that are designed for time trialing are lighter. They use fewer spokes and have an aerodynamic design. They can get away with being lighter because they generally don't encounter the same amount of varied or rough terrain that a road bike does. Other wheel options include a disk, deep dish, and trispoke.

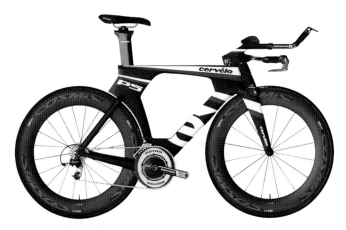

**Figure 13.4** Time-trialing bike.
Photo courtesy of Cervélo Cycles

A disk wheel is heavier than a spoked wheel, but it offers a big aerodynamic advantage. Both the disk and trispoke wheel are generally made of carbon fiber. With the carbon fiber disk wheel, an added bonus is that it sounds really cool when you shift gears. Many things must be taken into consideration when deciding on the proper wheel for an event. Climbs and heavy crosswinds are better served by the lighter spoked wheel; flat courses with front or tailwinds favor the disk.

TT bikes have a wide range of gearing, but sometimes they only have rear shifting capability. Having only a single chainring in the front cuts down on wind resistance and weight. Obviously, if you are riding on varied terrain with climbs, it's worthwhile to sacrifice the drag for a second chainring in the front. The shifting levers are mounted on the tips of the aerobars so you don't have to change your aero position to shift.

TT bikes are fun to ride and just downright cool. But, if you're deciding on a TT bike, I would suggest that you have another bike to make sure you can cover all your riding needs. The TT bike is a highly specialized piece of equipment. Even if your primary reason for riding is to participate in triathlons, you likely want to have a standard road bike as well. You can use the road bike for general training and for riding with groups of people.

## Cyclocross Bikes

These are old-school European machines. Picture muddy racers flinging their frames over their shoulders as they run over obstacles in the rain and snow. It's like a steeplechase for bikes! Cyclocross bikes are a ton of fun, and many people are using them as all-around bikes. Some of the most enjoyable rides are on cyclocross bikes because they allow you to flow between dirt trails and pavement.

At first glance, the frame looks like a road racing frame with the same downward angled (or drop) handlebars. However, a closer look reveals a stouter frame and a more relaxed geometry (meaning a shallower angle at the seat tube and headtube). Rather than the smooth, pavement-specific tires, these bikes are equipped with wider tires that have knobby treads (figure 13.5). The wheel size is the same as a road bike, 700c. The gearing ratios are different than a road bike. They have a wider range on the easier end, allowing you to climb in aggressive, dirty, and steep terrain.

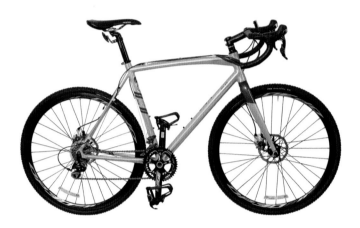

**Figure 13.5** Cyclocross bike.

## Touring Bikes and Hybrids

Ready to go on a bike trip? The touring bike is made for comfort and carrying loads. It has thicker tubing, and the geometry is designed for comfort rather than performance. The more relaxed geometry makes the bike less twitchy when descending. This is especially important when loaded down with camping gear.

Touring bikes usually have drop handlebars, and they come equipped with gearing that allows you to climb and cruise even when your panniers are full. (Panniers are the bags that hang off the racks of your bike.) The frame is fitted with eyelets for attaching front and rear racks or fenders. As with a road bike, the wheels are 700c, but they are comparatively wider, usually ranging from 28 to 35 millimeters.

Hybrids are great for commuters or townies (bikes for cruising or running errands around town). They come in a variety of styles and looks. Their primary purpose is to offer you a comfortable ride over moderate distances. They usually have gearing, either with a standard derailleur or an internal geared rear hub. Like touring bikes, hybrids are usually designed to carry racks and attach fenders. So many options are available that it really comes down to personal style preference and the feel of the bike when you ride it.

# Choosing Accessories

Now come all the extras. There is nearly a limitless supply of bike accessories. I'm always flipping through magazines and admiring the various items that will "enhance" my riding. But you should make sure that you take care of the important items first. Helmet, shoes, and pedals should be highest on your list. Then a good pair of shorts. The rest can fall into place over time. The following are descriptions of some of the most important items.

## Helmet

A helmet should be the first accessory that you buy. As an emergency physician and previous bike racer, I can attest to the lifesaving attributes of a high-quality helmet. Standing up after a crash, having your helmet crumble, and then being coherent enough to appreciate the damage is an eye-opening experience.

The purpose of a helmet is to dissipate the peak energy of an impact. Most helmets provide this protection with expanded polystyrene (EPS), the foam substance (resembling the material of a foam cooler) inside the helmet. When your head experiences an impact, the EPS absorbs the energy by crushing and cracking throughout the helmet. Most helmets meet minimal safety standards, but to be on the safe side, you should check for the CPSP sticker on the inside. This means that the helmet was inspected and cleared by the U.S. Consumer Product Safety Commission.

Your helmet should be light and comfortable. Wear it on every ride. If professional racers can tolerate a helmet in the intense heat and effort of racing up L'Alpe d'Huez in the Tour de France, then there is no doubt that you can tolerate it on a training ride. If you have a good helmet, wearing it should become second nature. You should never have to give it a second thought after you strap it to your head.

Make sure your helmet fits properly. Visit your local bike shop and have them help you find your correct size. Look for a helmet that has some sort of ratchet system to ensure a snug yet comfortable fit. Make sure you wear the helmet over your forehead. You'll often see riders, especially kids, with their helmets sitting back on the crown of their head like a yarmulke. That won't protect you in a front impact.

Remember, once you crash or damage a helmet, it is no longer useful. By design, the foam dissipates energy by destroying itself. Therefore, after an impact, the foam is "used up." Your brain is valuable enough that you shouldn't take the risk of using a helmet that won't protect you in a fall.

## Shoes and Pedals

Professional cyclists are obsessive about their shoes. Hop on any team bus before a race and you'll see riders cleaning their shoes with alcohol wipes!

The proper shoe is dependent on the type of bike you'll be riding. Road shoes have extremely stiff soles. They're made of carbon fiber, titanium, or plastic. The stiffness efficiently transfers all the energy from your leg to the pedal and cranks. The stiffness also allows for better control of the bike. The cleat is usually large in order to provide good solid contact with the pedal. It sticks out from the shoe and makes walking difficult.

Mountain bike and cross shoes are designed as a compromise between performance stiffness on the bike and the ability to walk or run in rough terrain off the bike. This is accomplished, in part, by having a recessed cleat. The cleat is recessed into the sole of a treaded shoe.

Touring shoes are the most flexible of the bunch. They are designed to provide the most comfort when walking off of the bike. They have recessed cleats like the shoes for mountain and cross bikes. At first glance, they look more like a tennis shoe or hiking boot than a road racing shoe.

Regardless of the shoe type, comfort is paramount. Make sure your shoe fits well. Every shoemaker has unique characteristics (i.e., wide, narrow, high arch, low arch). Try on numerous pairs to get a feel for what works best on your foot.

Try out the various latching systems on different models. Shoelaces are becoming less and less common. Many shoes use Velcro or a ratcheted system (like a ski boot) to really lock your foot in place. Foot movement in the shoe can cause blisters and soreness. It also bleeds off power that could be transferred to the bike.

Old racing bikes came equipped with toe clips and leather straps. People who still use this system may get high style points for being retro, but the newer clipless pedals do a better job. Clipless pedals lock the shoe onto the pedal using a binding system. If you twist your foot to the side, your shoe will release. This may feel a little threatening at first, but once you do it a few times, you'll get the hang of popping your shoe in and out of the pedal.

A wide range of pedal choices are also available (figure 13.6). Road bike pedals offer a solid platform with good ground clearance so you can pedal deep into a corner. Mountain and cross bike systems allow for entry and exit even when the pedal is full of mud and debris. Touring pedals may offer not only a binding system, but also a standard pedal platform so you can ride the bike with or without your specific cycling shoe.

Clipless systems offer various ranges of float. Float is the amount of angular movement your foot has while locked into the pedal. A fixed pedal-cleat system has no movement, whereas a free-float system allows your foot to move about a vertical axis drawn through the ball of your foot. I recommend a system that allows movement because it reduces the risk of poor alignment

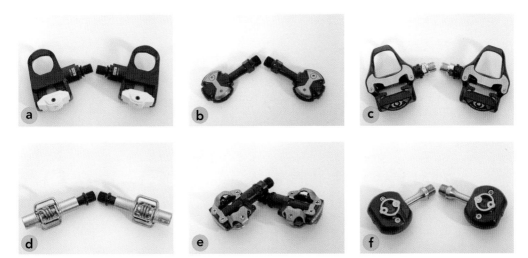

**Figure 13.6** Road pedals: *(a)* Look, *(b)* Speedplay, *(c)* Shimano; mountain pedals: *(d)* Crankbrothers eggbeater, *(e)* Shimano SPD, *(f)* Speedplay.

and subsequent injury. The amount of float will be mentioned in the pedal marketing description. Your local bike shop can show you the various pedal systems and help you figure out what is best for your situation.

When purchasing shoes and cleats, you should be sure to consult a salesperson in order to make sure that the items are compatible. A mountain bike shoe does not work with a road pedal, nor does a road shoe work with a mountain bike pedal.

## Shorts

Proper clothing makes riding more comfortable and enjoyable. When starting out, most people are concerned about keeping their backside comfortable on the saddle. This can be greatly aided by wearing a good pair of cycling shorts. If you ask professional cyclists to identify the most important clothing items, they will likely say shorts and shoes. This is because these items provide the major contact points with the bike.

Cycling shorts offer a padded chamois typically made of a moisture-absorbing synthetic material (figure 13.7). Originally, all chamois were leather, but technology has now stepped to the forefront. You should buy gender-specific shorts because men and women have different points of irritation and chaffing. A good chamois is definitely worth the money.

Most cycling shorts are form fitting and made of a stretchy material. The tight fit keeps your thighs and butt from rubbing on the saddle. Shorts come in a standard style with a waistband or a bib style that has straps that go over each shoulder like suspenders. Professionals and serious riders wear bibs because they are more comfortable if riding for extended periods. If

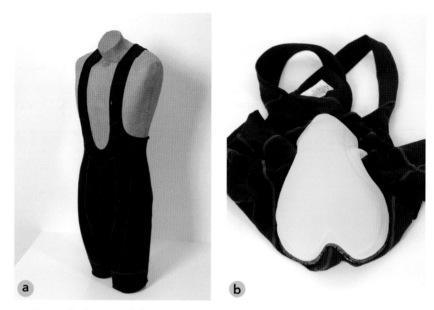

**Figure 13.7** Bib shorts and chamois.

you don't like the tight look of standard cycling shorts, you can buy a pair of baggy shorts with a cycling chamois short hidden inside.

Don't wear underwear underneath your cycling shorts. This will defeat the purpose and design of the shorts. You should have at least two pairs of shorts because it's important that you wash your shorts and chamois after every ride. This keeps bacteria out of the chamois and decreases your risk of developing saddle sores.

## Jerseys

Cycling jerseys have come a long way from the original wool models seen in black-and-white cycling photos. Today, jerseys are made of technical fibers that wick away moisture and promote breathability. They are form fitting to cut down on wind resistance, and they have pockets in the back to store food, clothing, or any accessories you may need on a ride. Newer jerseys have either full-zip or three-quarter-zip fronts. The full-zip fronts are easier to vent and remove if needed. Jerseys come in various fabrics, sleeve lengths, and thickness to best accommodate different riding conditions. Layering is a good idea because you can adapt to changing weather.

## Clothing Accessories

Numerous clothing accessories are available. After you spend time on the bike, you'll start to discover your personal preferences for gear. Here are a few of the more common items:

- **Gloves:** Riding with gloves is always a good idea. Gloves cushion the contact with the bars and help keep your hands safe if you happen to lay the bike down in a crash. Fingerless gloves are the most common. They allow you to still have dexterity to work zippers, eat, and control shifters and brake levers. Some mountain bikers prefer full-finger versions for increased protection from the rough terrain. Obviously, if you ride in cold weather, you'll want to purchase thermal gloves. Lobster gloves are great at keeping your fingers warm if they're prone to freezing up in chilly conditions.

- **Arm and leg warmers:** These are great additions to your cycling kit. They are extremely versatile. They're easy to get on and off, and they're light so they can slip into the rear pockets of your jersey. You should use arm and leg warmers as part of your layering system.

- **Tights:** On cold days, you may want to wear a pair of tights. Some tights come with a chamois attached, and some are designed to slip over your regular cycling shorts. The weather in your area will dictate whether you need tights, but for most riders, leg warmers may do the trick.

- **Jackets:** All kinds of cycling jackets are available, ranging from thin wind-breaking jackets to thick thermals. A good breathable rain jacket is nice to have at your disposal. Again, the weather you plan on riding in will dictate what you need. As mentioned earlier, layering may be a better option than wearing a single thick jacket.

- **Glasses:** Glasses are an essential component of your cycling kit. They protect your eyes from wind, glare, ultraviolet (UV) rays, insects, and dirt and debris thrown up by cars and other riders. Make sure the glasses are light and offer enough wraparound protection. Some glasses have lenses that are interchangeable. Even on overcast or rainy days, you should be sure to wear eye protection. You can get different lenses depending on the conditions: shaded, clear, yellow, amber, and pink.

## Hydration Options

Proper hydration is essential during your rides. Water bottle cages are the classic and still preferred method for carrying water. They'll accommodate both short 12-ounce bottles and tall 16-ounce bottles. Having two water bottle cages on your bike is a good option in case you do a long ride or it is particularly hot outside. Cages come in all shapes and metal types—plastic, steel, aluminum, titanium, and carbon fiber. Don't get too carried away with spending a fortune on a water bottle cage. A race has never been won because someone had a lighter water bottle carrier.

Some riders prefer hydration packs. These can be advantageous for mountain and cross bike rides. There are times when the terrain limits the rider's ability to reach down and grab a bottle. The hydration pack solves this problem so that the rider can drink on the go, even if the trail is technical. You should keep as much weight off your back as possible. The riding position already strains your lower back, and anything that limits the stress is advisable.

## Repair Kits

You should be prepared to handle minor malfunctions during a ride. This includes being able to change a tire and make simple repairs. To do this, you need to bring a spare tube, a tube repair kit, and a pump. Some people prefer $CO_2$ canisters rather than a pump. The advantage is that they are small and they fill the tire with air quickly. The disadvantage is that each canister gives you only one shot at inflating your tire. If you mess up the connection between the tube and the canister, or if you get more than one flat tire, you may find yourself stranded. If you decide to go with the canister option, make sure you carry at least two.

You should also have some sort of combination tool (figure 13.8). Depending on the one you purchase, the tool may include hex wrenches, a screwdriver, a spoke wrench, and a chain tool. You never know when you may need to tighten a loose seat or handlebar, adjust a cleat, or pop off a broken link in your chain.

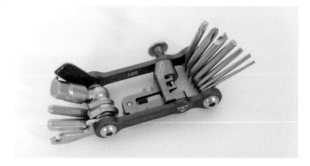

**Figure 13.8** Combination tool.

This chapter provided information to help you become well equipped to go for a ride. You should browse through magazines and bike shops to get a good idea of what is out there and how various products will suit your riding style and goals. Remember to focus on the big-ticket items first. The cool trinkets will always be available, but don't get sidetracked from the basics until you're outfitted to ride safely and comfortably.

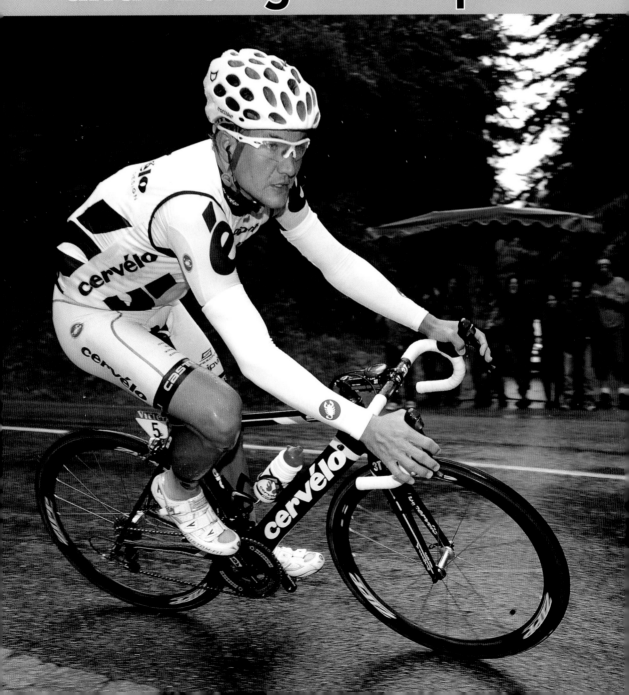

# Refining Bike Fit
# and Riding Techniques

**This** chapter focuses on proper rider position, riding technique, and bike-handling skills. The importance of a good bike fit cannot be over-emphasized. Comfort, power, and injury avoidance all depend, in part, on your body's alignment when riding. This chapter takes you through the key measurements in situating yourself correctly. Whether you decide to have a professional fit or do it yourself, after reading this chapter, you'll know the ins and outs of what to look for when sizing and adjusting your frame setup. There's good and bad technique when you ride. In this chapter, you'll learn the best way to handle your bike, pedal efficiently, and use all the gear ratios at your disposal. Finally, the chapter ends with some good exercises that will pay dividends once you get on the road or ride in groups.

## Frame Size

A classic road frame has a top tube that is parallel with the ground. These frames are fairly square—meaning that unless it is a custom frame, the top tube and the seat tube are close to the same length. Over the past decade, compact frames have become much more popular. They have a slanted top tube that is higher in the front at the head tube than in the back where the top tube meets the seat tube. They're "compact" because the triangle inside the top, down, and seat tubes is smaller than on a classic frame. The advantage is less weight and increased stiffness. Sizing for compact frames is simplified: small, medium, and large. Manufacturers customize them by changing the stem length, stem angle, and seat tube length.

For classic frames, sizes are usually based on the height of the seat tube. Depending on the manufacturer, the size is measured in either centimeters or inches. Usually, road bikes are measured in centimeters (e.g., 56 centimeters), and mountain bikes in inches (e.g., 18 inches). Other manufactures size bikes as small, medium, and large. A general rule when sizing a classic frame is to use your stand-over height. You should have 1 to 2 inches (2.5 to 5.1 cm) of clearance between the top tube and your crotch when standing over the top tube. For compact frames (both road and mountain bike), the manufacturer will have a sizing chart to best fit you to the frame size based on your height and inseam length.

## Cycling Position

Cycling position isn't just about looking good on your bike. It's about performance. Have you noticed how pros look so relaxed and aero when they're riding? It comes from years of training and honing their position.

The following sections will give you a good starting measurement. There is no way to provide every cyclist with the perfect position merely by writing down instructions. But, if you follow these instructions, you'll have a great fit to start with. You can then slowly tweak your position until you find the ultimate power, comfort, and aerodynamics.

## Shoe Position (Cleat Position)

The first step in your fit is to set up your cycling shoes properly. If you are serious about your riding, you should use clipless pedals and cycling-specific shoes. To set up the cleat on the shoe, pay attention to how you walk and stand. Do you walk with your toes inward or outward (pigeon-toed or duck-footed)? You want to replicate a similar angle with your foot when placing the cleat. Many people try to make their cleats align perfectly to the forward moving direction of the bike; instead, you should match the cleat angle with your foot position when walking and standing. The cleat should also be placed so the spindle of the pedal goes directly under the ball of your foot.

## Saddle Position

Saddle position has three components: seat height, fore-aft position, and seat angle (figure 14.1). All three of these are important to getting the most out of your pedaling motion. Muscle fibers have an optimal firing position. Setting up your seat properly will help you efficiently use your power. Correct position will also help alleviate undue pressure points, soreness, and chafing. The following information will guide you when setting up your bike at home. You should have a friend help you make the adjustments. If you get a professional fit, you can use the information provided to help you better understand the adjustments as the person dials in your setup.

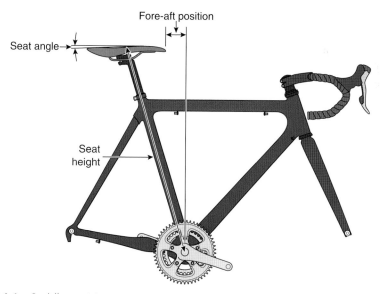

**Figure 14.1**   Saddle position.

- **Seat height:** Place your bike in a trainer (make sure you slightly raise the front wheel to simulate a completely flat road) and sit squarely on the seat. Before you clip in to your pedals, adjust your seat so your heel just touches the pedal. This is a good starting point. Now clip your shoes in to the pedals. When your crank is in the 6 o'clock position, you want to have a slight bend at the knee (see figure 14.2a). Make slight adjustments up and down to find the most comfortable locations. As you pedal in the trainer, you want your hips to remain steady. If they are rocking back and forth, then you need to lower your seat a bit more. Be sure the seat post isn't overextended. Seat posts usually have a clearly marked line that should not be exceeded when extending the post out of the frame.

- **Fore-aft position:** The fore-aft position starts with the cleat on your shoe. The cleat should be adjusted so that the spindle of the pedal lines up just under the ball of your foot. The angle of the cleat should mimic the position of your foot when you stand at rest (e.g., pigeon-toed, duck-footed). Next, you'll need to set up a plum line. This is basically a pointed weight on the end of a string. You can get this at any hardware store. Get on the bike and clip in to your pedals. Adjust your crank to the horizontal 3 o'clock position. Hold the top of the string over your kneecap and watch where the pointed weight falls on your foot. (See figure 14.2b.) Move your seat fore or aft so that the pointed weight points directly over the spindle of the pedal. After you dial this in, you'll have to go back to the seat height and make minor adjustments.

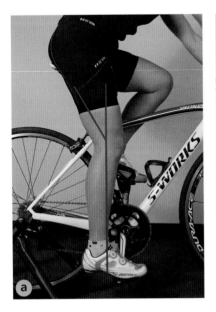
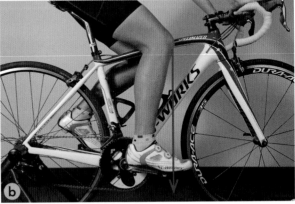

**Figure 14.2** Proper saddle position. *(a)* The correct height will result in a slight bend of your knee. *(b)* For-aft position is determined by dropping a plumb line from your knee through the spindle of your pedal.

- **Seat angle:** A good starting point is to lay a level over the top of the saddle and make it parallel with the ground. After you ride a bit and have the other positions properly adjusted, see how you feel while riding. You shouldn't feel excessive pressure from the nose of the saddle in your crotch. You also shouldn't feel as if you are falling forward onto the handlebar. Any adjustment to the angle should be slight. Big changes can cause big problems!

Fitting your saddle can be a tedious process. Each adjustment of one of the parameters will cause slight changes in the other two. With each successive change, the distances will become smaller and smaller until you have your position totally honed. After you complete the measurements in the next section, come back to your saddle height to make sure nothing has changed.

## Handlebar Position and Reach

Proper handlebar position and reach depend on the type of riding you'll be doing. Whether you're on a road, mountain, touring, or hybrid bike, your position is a trade-off between aerodynamics, comfort, and control. The farther forward your position, the more aerodynamic it will be. But a forward position puts increased strain on your arms and back. If you are extremely far forward, you may have issues with control because your weight is so far over the front wheel.

With your saddle properly adjusted, your reach is controlled by three factors: stem height, stem length, and stem angle (figure 14.3). Let's start with stem height. On a road bike, the stem height should be even with or

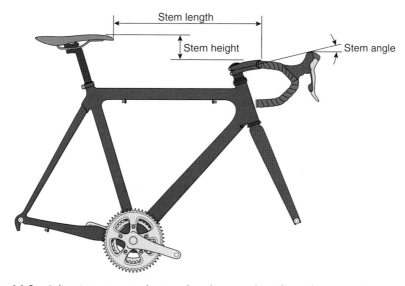

**Figure 14.3**   Adjusting your reach: stem height, stem length, and stem angle.

slightly lower than your seat (racers have it much lower than their seat). If you have a bad back or you are riding a touring or hybrid bike, you'll want to raise your stem until comfortable. As mentioned, as you raise the height, you'll increase your wind resistance. For the most part, mountain bikes need less adjustment. The best plan is to ride with whatever stem the bike comes with. Over time, if you think that you are too far forward or too upright, you can visit your local bike shop to try different stem options.

Stem length and stem angle go hand in hand. As you adjust your position, pay attention to how far you extend over the front wheel. To size a road bike, you should have a slight bend in your elbows when on the hoods. The front stem length and angle are correct if the horizontal part of your handlebar obstructs your view of the front hub. For a touring, hybrid, or cross bike, the front hub should be slightly in front of the horizontal handlebar (figure 14.4).

Every time you adjust your position, you'll need to take the bike out for a ride to see how it feels. Some initial discomfort is normal while your body adjusts, but if you continue to be uncomfortable, develop persistent back or neck pain, or have hand numbness, you'll need to go back and adjust your position.

For professional bike fits, various options are available, and these can vary greatly in price. Some are done manually, similar to what has been described

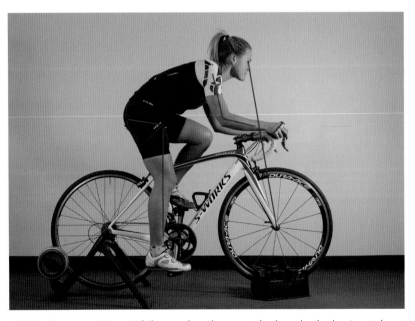

**Figure 14.4** Proper position. While your hands are on the hoods, the horizontal part of the handlebar should obstruct the view of your front hub.

in this section. More advanced technology using video and computer imaging evaluates your position while you are moving. This helps ensure that you're as efficient as possible. Don't be alarmed if a professional fit sets you up slightly different than what's described here. The information provided is a good starting point, but it must be adapted to each individual.

Regardless of how you obtain your original fit, if you spend a lot of time on the bike, you'll start to feel where you would like to make adjustments. Always make small changes. Drastic changes will lead to undue stress on your body.

# Riding Technique

You want to get the most out of your ride. Proper riding technique improves efficiency and performance. Cycling may have seemed simple enough once you mastered the whole balance aspect as a kid, but there are a lot of nuances that can designate you as a performance rider rather than an average Joe.

## Efficiency and Pedaling Motion

Next time you ride, focus on your pedaling motion. Are you smooth? At which part of the pedal stroke do you apply power to the pedals? Does your body rock back and forth on the saddle? Thinking about the way you pedal can vastly improve your performance. Any wasted or inefficient movement multiplied by the number of times you turn the cranks on a ride can start to add up.

Many beginner cyclists stomp on the pedals, applying pressure only on the downstroke. Focus on keeping both legs working for the entire revolution. Coaches use the phrase "pedaling in circles." Some researchers also refer to pedaling in triangles. This may sound strange, but studies have shown that some elite riders in fact apply pressure that is consistent with the shape of a triangle: pushing down and forward, pulling back at the bottom of the pedaling arc, and pulling upward to the top of the pedal stroke. Whatever works mentally for you is fine. The point is that you want to apply pressure consistently. Don't waste half of the pedal stroke letting your leg idly stand by. Even worse, don't make one leg lift the weight of the other!

Some riders have switched from a circular front chainring to an oval shape. The idea behind the design is to minimize the amount of time in your rotational "dead spot"—usually the top and bottom of the pedal stroke. The oval theoretically changes the effective number of teeth in the chainring. For example, on the downstroke, when you have the most power, the oval acts as if it's a 56-tooth cog. This generates more power. However, at the bottom of the stroke, when your motion is the weakest, the oval acts as though there are only 51 teeth, better adapting to the weaker pull of your leg.

It is up to you whether you choose to use an oval or circular ring. The important thing is to focus more on applying smooth consistent pressure throughout your pedaling rotation. This will ensure that you're getting the most out of every revolution.

As your foot rotates around the pedal stroke, you should also think about your heel position and the fluidity of your leg movement. Avoid jerky or big movements. Smoothly move through your downstroke and slightly drop your heel. As you pass to the backside of the circle and start to elevate the crank, move your heel upward. A secret to achieving smooth pedaling technique is to ride a fixed gear in the off-season, focusing on smooth pedaling circles. Remember, excess movement wastes energy. Take note of the pros. Watch how smoothly they pedal, even at a fast rpm.

## Gearing and Cadence

Unless you're riding a fixed-gear or single-speed bike, your bike is equipped with a transmission, or gear system. This allows you to control your pedaling rpm (revolutions per minute) over varied terrain. By using various combinations of front and rear chainrings, you have a large range of gear ratios to choose from when you encounter varying riding conditions.

If you multiply the number of front chainrings by the number of rear cogs, you'll get the total number of gears. However, these are not all functional. Try to keep your chain tracking fairly straight along the direction of forward motion. Don't "cross over" by putting the chain on the largest outside ring in the front and the largest inside cog on the rear hub. Angling the chain can overstress it and cause breakage. Also, some efficiency is lost by not having the chain track along the direction of motion.

If you want to get technical, there are gear ratio calculators online that allow you to calculate your bike's gearing. But for now, let's look at some general concepts. The number of teeth on a chainring or cog determines its size. When referring to a road bike, for example, people will say, "I ride a 52-38." This means that they have a 52-tooth large chainring and a 38-tooth small chainring. The same applies for the rear hub. When people say, "I ride a 23-11," they are stating the full range of teeth on their largest and smallest rear cogs.

The biggest gear ratio is when your chain is on the large front chainring (most teeth) and the small cog (fewest teeth) on the rear hub. Your smallest gear ratio is just the opposite—fewest teeth in the front and most teeth in the rear.

It takes practice to use your gears fluidly and frequently. Just as your car is constantly shifting, you should frequently adjust your gearing based on the terrain, wind, road conditions, and level of fatigue. Don't get stuck riding in one or two gears. You've spent good, hard-earned money on a nice bike. Use it for all it's worth!

# Effect of rpm on Efficiency

Your rpm (revolutions per minute) plays a big role in your efficiency. For every individual, there is a unique tempo that will best utilize his physiology. Riding hard is a constant balance between oxygenation and ventilation in the lungs and between energy production and waste management at the muscle. By changing your cadence, you control the rate at which these processes occur.

In the lab, a rider's heart rate, power output, and even lactic acid production can be monitored moment to moment as the rider shifts from one gear to another. It is amazing that just the right cadence can increase speed while making little change in heart rate and lactic acid production. This is the sweet spot for a hard effort.

A good experiment is to find a climb and test yourself. Try climbing in a hard gear (bigger gear ratio), and then, once recovered, do it again in an easier gear (smaller gear ratio). See if your performance changes. Try to find the gear ratio that makes you feel the most comfortable while at the same time preserving or increasing your speed.

If you have a home trainer, a heart rate monitor, and a power meter, you can mimic the lab experiment. Perform interval training (see chapter 7) and record your heart rate and power output at various cadences (by changing your rpm). See if you can find your own sweet spot.

Professional riders climb at a brisk cadence. When professional riders are on form, they will spin at between 90 and 95 rpm in a stage race. This minimizes the wear and tear on the muscles, keeping them fresh for the next day of hard effort. They also like the fast cadence because they can better accelerate when the race surges. If you are in too big of a gear, you can "burn out your clutch" by trying to jump on an attack.

If you have trouble riding up a climb at a quick cadence, slowly work into it. As with everything in training, you should take baby steps. Slowly but surely your technique, form, and conditioning will improve until you're climbing like a pro!

Bicycle gears allow you to control your cadence. Part of becoming a skilled cyclist is knowing which cadence gives you the best performance on a given terrain. During a hard effort, you'll start to feel the pain in both your legs and lungs. Always try to match your leg burn to your lung burn. This can be accomplished by changing your cadence. As sadistic as it sounds, your goal should be to equally distribute the suffering. If your lungs hurt more than your legs, decrease your cadence and push a bigger gear. If your legs burn more than your lungs, shift into an easier gear and increase the rpm.

It is difficult to actually count your cadence while riding. If you're interested in training with cadence, some affordable bike computers come with this option. Be sure to check for this feature on the packaging before you make a purchase. Most power meters come with a cadence measure. The readout gives you both your power and cadence at the same time. You are able to see the moment-to-moment change of power as you shift gears to vary your rpm.

## Bike-Handling Skills

Riding on the road means that you always have to be alert and ready to take evasive action. The better your bike-handling skills, the more likely you'll come out unscathed. As with anything, practice makes perfect. It's better to work on handling skills before you need them, rather than wait for an emergency. Being calm and confident on the bike may get you out of a bad situation. Even if you ride alone, you can't always predict what's around the next corner or what the car just ahead of you will do. If you ride in packs, you'll need to be even more comfortable on the bike because of the proximity of other riders.

Following are a few exercises that may come in handy. Find a quiet area without cars or obstacles so you can focus your attention on the exercise rather than on obstacles. Whatever type of bike you're riding (road, mountain, cross, hybrid, or touring), all of these exercises are applicable and valuable.

- **Wheelies**—Many of us mastered the wheelie as a kid on our BMX bikes. Feeling comfortable popping the front wheel can save you if you're about to roll over an obstacle. Settle yourself on the pedals, and when comfortable, yank up on the handlebar. Start small and slowly build up. Robbie McEwen is a professional road racer famous for coming over the finish line riding a wheelie on his racing bike.

- **Bunny hops**—I've been saved many times by the bunny hop, and that's not hyperbole. This is an excellent skill to master. You should practice a bunny hop until you have no problem clearing a curb or pothole. While rolling, pull up with both feet and hands at the same time. Both of the wheels should come off the ground at the same time.

- **Tight circles**—Find a parking space or other marker in the pavement. While riding at slow speed, work on making as tight a circle as possible without falling over. Don't forget to do this drill in both directions. The purpose is to give you a good feel for your bike while also enhancing your balance. This exercise will help you feel comfortable in tight spaces and in packs.

- **Rapid braking**—Accelerate to a sprint and then coast. Rapidly apply your brakes to stop as quickly as possible without skidding. Remember that the majority of your stopping power comes from your front brake. The tricky part is that if you overapply the front brake, you can flip or "endo." This drill will help you get a feel for how quickly you can stop. It will also help you learn the proper technique for rapidly decelerating without losing control.

- **Track stands**—You've likely seen a bike rider doing this at a traffic stop. Make sure you've mastered popping out of your pedals before attempting this exercise. You want to feel confident that you can abort if you start to fall over. Like the other drills, this hones your sense of balance and connection to the bike. Hold your hands on the brakes, turn your wheel to one side, and stand on the pedals. You may have to rock back and forth just a bit to maintain your balance.

- **Cornering**—Pick a smooth, sweeping corner without obstacles or debris. Come into the corner, slow at first and then more quickly. Feel your bike lean over. Get comfortable driving through the corner. Remember that you can't pedal through the corner because your pedal may clip the ground. Focus on driving the ball of your outside foot through the bottom of the pedal with the foot in the 6 o'clock position on the crank. You'll get a feel for how much grip you have coming into a corner. Remember, try not to brake while sweeping through the corner. Traction is in limited supply. If you brake, you'll be using up some of your grip to slow the bike and some to keep the tire from slipping out. It's better to use your traction for keeping the tire on the pavement.

# Pack Riding

Riding in an echelon, a paceline, or a big pack is one of the thrills of cycling. A group of riders can always motor faster than a solo effort. But riding in proximity to other riders does increase the potential hazard. Here are a few tips to help you avoid unnecessary problems:

- Always leave a bit of space, even when drafting. You'll still get good wind protection even if you're a foot or two behind the rider in front of you.

- Never cross wheels with the rider in front of you. That way, if the rider makes a rapid move or tries to avoid an obstacle, she won't clip your wheel.

- Communicate with the other riders. If you see an obstacle in the road, make sure the riders behind you know what's coming. They might not be able to see around you.

- Hold your line. Don't make any sudden movements. Riders expect that you'll keep tracking along your current course and speed. If you need to make a move, talk and let the other riders know what you're doing.
- Keep a steady tempo. If riding in a paceline (a single-file line of riders), you should push a slightly bigger gear than you would if you were riding that speed alone. This will smooth out your ride. Also, avoid touching your brakes unless absolutely necessary. Try to control your speed with your power output.

Having the proper fit on your bike is extremely important. You're a performance cyclist, and having the proper fit will improve your efficiency and power output. It will also give you the best control and bike handling. You'll obviously improve your skills while logging the miles of your training, but it is always worthwhile to spend a little time specifically working on your bike-handling skills. You'll ride better, descend faster, and avoid potential hazards because you took the time to feel totally comfortable on your bike.

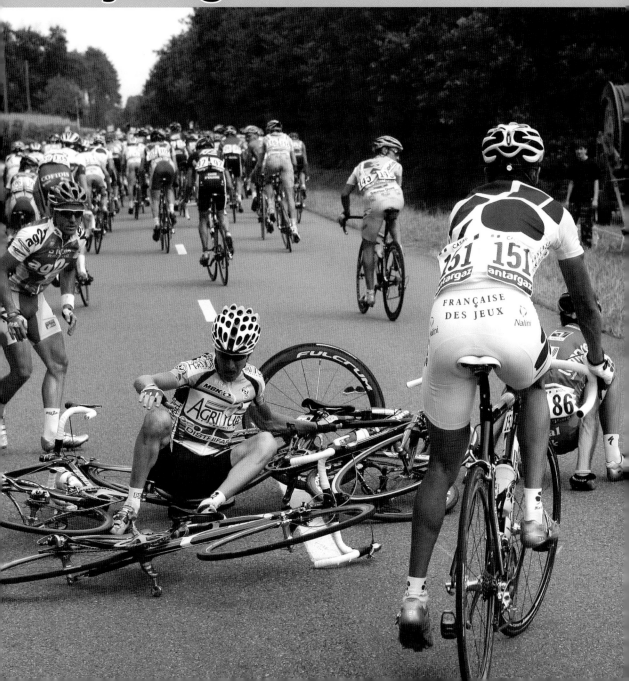

# 15

# Dealing With Common Cycling Problems

**As** mentioned numerous times in this book, cycling is a fantastic sport. It has so much to offer. You work your cardiovascular system while also getting the thrill of experiencing and exploring the outdoors. It is a low-impact, body-friendly sport. When other sports break your body down, cycling is often written into the rehabilitation program because of its smooth motion and ease on your joints.

However, like any endurance sport, if you do it enough (or overdo it), cycling can cause you to develop aches and pains. If you don't address the problems early, they can become nagging problems and force you to seek medical attention.

Cycling injuries come in two main categories: trauma and overuse or strain injuries. The first is obvious, and all cyclists hope to keep the rubber side down on their rides. Nobody wants to crash, but if you do find yourself on the ground, you need to understand acute care. The second—more insidious—group of injuries comes on slowly and can be more debilitating than a crash. In this chapter, you'll learn about acute care procedures. In addition, the chapter addresses common cycling ailments that may develop over time and provides information that will direct your recovery.

The first key to taking care of cycling injuries is to be smart and use your head. If you crash or start to develop aches and pains, you need to rest. It is better to address things right away. If you are having knee problems, take some time off the bike. Think about why you may be having the pain: Did you torque or twist the knee? Did something happen off the bike? Did you buy new equipment or change your position? Think through all the possible reasons that you could be feeling pain.

Remember that you're in cycling for the long haul, so don't ignore symptoms when they arrive. Take a break and rest before your symptoms worsen. Pain is your body's way of telling you that something is wrong. Listen to your body's cues before real damage is done.

Here are some general rules for cycling injuries:

1. Address the problem promptly.
2. Have a professional check out your problem. Obviously, if you crash, this may mean a trip to the emergency department or your doctor. If you have ongoing aches and pains, you should visit a sports medical center or your primary doctor for advice.
3. Rest. Don't be a hero. It is better to take a short rest now rather than an unavoidable long break later.
4. Establish a plan for avoiding the same problem in the future.

# RICE

When you have aches and pains, or after a trauma, remember the acronym RICE. By employing RICE therapy, you'll get back on the road as soon as possible. The sooner you start to take care of your problem, the shorter the amount of time you'll be off the bike.

- **Rest**—If it hurts, your body is telling you to take a break. Listen to the cues your body is giving you, and give yourself a chance to heal.
- **Ice**—Crushed ice, frozen corn, or frozen peas are great for molding to the area of injury. Apply ice over a thin fabric protecting the skin. For best results, apply ice in a pattern of 15 minutes on followed by 15 minutes off.
- **Compression**—If able, use an elastic wrap to hold the ice in place. This will help limit the swelling.
- **Elevation**—Keep the injured area above the level of your heart. Merely lying down may not be enough. Look at the level of your heart above the ground. Try to keep the injury at a higher point in space.

# Road Rash

We all suffered the occasional abrasion as kids. And if you've ridden a bike for any length of time, you've probably had a close encounter with the ramifications of friction. *Road rash* sounds so much "cooler" than *abrasion*, so as a cyclist, at least you have that going for you.

The primary issue with road rash is infection control and scarring. The first order of business is to thoroughly clean your wounds as soon as possible. This not only limits the risk of infection, but it also makes the pain a bit more manageable. If you clean the wounds promptly, you'll still have some of the adrenaline flowing, and this helps you deal with pain.

Remove any big pieces of grass, rocks, or other foreign material. Ideally, you should flow clean water over the wound. The easiest way to do this is in the shower. If you can't get to a shower for a while, you can poke holes in the lids of plastic water bottles and then locally shower the abrasions.

Next, clean the wound using gauze or a clean washcloth and very diluted soapy water. Do this gently but try to get out any debris that is stuck in the wound. Do not scrub the wound aggressively because this can cause more damage to the tissue—not to mention make grown adults cry like little babies!

Avoid using hydrogen peroxide or cleaning solutions such as Hibiclens. Strong cleaning solutions can injure the remaining cells at the border of the wound and slow healing. Again, diluted soapy water is your best option.

Once you've cleaned the wound, apply a thin layer of antibiotic ointment. Neosporin and bacitrin are common and easy to find. Bacitracin is a better option because some people are allergic to one of the components of Neosporin. Dress the wound with nonstick gauze pads. This is key, because if you use plain gauze you'll be cursing yourself when you try to change the dressing and it won't come off of the wound. If you do have problems removing the dressing, try soaking it in the shower or bath. This will help release the gauze pad from the healing tissue.

Leave the wound open as much as possible. Obviously, you may have to work or go out in public, but when you're home, try to open the abrasion up to the air. This will help with healing and cut down on the fortune you'll be spending on gauze and medical supplies.

Wounds scar; there is no way around it. A ton of information is available on scar reduction. Different plastic surgeons have different techniques and products. Some recommend removing the scab, and others do not. I prefer to let the wound heal by scabbing and to remove the scab only when it is nearly falling off on its own. By far, the biggest factor in reducing scarring is keeping the wound out of the sun. This goes beyond the acute phase of the injury. The healing skin will continue to repair itself for months. A good rule is to keep the tissue covered (either with clothes or sunscreen) for at least the first 6 months.

Watch for signs of infection. Initially, the edges of the wound will be red from the acute trauma, and this is normal. However, if you notice that it starts to worsen in the days after the injury, have a professional check it out. Other signs of infection are increased pain, pus (white) discharge, red streaking away from the wound, and fever. If you are concerned about infection, see a doctor right away. The sooner you start treatment, the less the chance of complication, and the better off you'll be.

## Saddle Sores

Nobody likes to think or talk about saddle sores, but if you get serious about riding, they may be something that you'll have to deal with. First, let's differentiate between chafing and saddle sores. Chafing is the irritation that develops from friction, either from your clothes or saddle. This is easily treated by adjusting your equipment, taking a break, and using creams.

If you continue to ride on pressure points, you can sometimes develop a true saddle sore. These are inflammatory or infectious nodules that develop in hair follicles and sweat glands. Like with many things, avoidance is the best medicine. Cleanliness and proper clothing will go a long way toward making sure you don't have to deal with saddle sores. Wear well-fitting cycling shorts directly against your skin (no underwear). Make sure your saddle is right for you. Don't skimp on comfort for weight. I did that once and learned my lesson the hard way. I've ridden the same brand of seat now for over 10 years.

Don't hang out in your chamois (cycling shorts) after you complete your ride. Try to change into regular shorts as soon as possible, and better yet, take a quick shower. This is a big deal for professionals. They shower in the bus immediately after getting off the bike. If they have to go to the podium and can't shower, at a minimum they change out their shorts for a clean pair.

Make sure you clean your chamois well. Follow the manufacturer's directions. Immediately after washing your shorts, hang them out to dry. Don't let them sit wet or moist in the washing machine. This allows bacteria to breed.

Finally, use chamois cream. Numerous brands are on the market, and you'll have to find what works for you. DZ Nuts works well and is available in most bike shops.

## Neck Pain

Neck pain usually develops because of the prolonged hyperflexion from your riding position. During the off-season, you should work to strengthen and stretch your neck muscles. Start with range-of-motion exercises and then add subtle resistance exercises. Chapter 3 of *Cycling Anatomy* (Human Kinetics, 2009) includes numerous sample exercises. Remember that the shoulder and neck muscles cross over and are closely related; therefore, a good program will strengthen the entire shoulder and neck area.

At the beginning of the training year, ease into your rides. Slowly ramp up your time in the saddle. This will allow your neck muscles to adapt just like the rest of your physiology. Many cyclists get overly excited for the first weekend of good weather, and they immediately go on a monster ride. This sets them back a week or two.

If you develop neck pain during the season, you should take a few days off the bike. Make sure you do range-of-motion exercises. If your symptoms persist, you should see your health care provider. You may have to take a look at your position. Corrective options include raising or shortening your stem. You can also find a stem with a more vertical angle. Sometimes you can turn your stem upside down if that makes the position less aggressive.

## Hand and Wrist Pain

Ulnar neuropathy is a condition that causes numbness and tingling in your hand, often in your little and ring finger. It results from prolonged pressure on the ulnar nerve.

Some of the problem can be relieved with proper positioning. Take some pressure off your hands by shortening your reach. Decreasing the distance to the handlebars will reposition some of your weight onto your saddle. Follow the instructions in chapter 14 on positioning, or if you have the resources, get a professional bike fit. Local bike shops will likely have resources in your area.

Another simple solution is to wear padded cycling gloves. Gel-filled gloves not only reduce the direct pressure by distributing the weight over your entire hand, they also dampen the vibration that comes through the bars. This is also where some frame materials beat the others in terms of comfort. For example, aluminum frames transmit much more of the road vibration than a steel or titanium frame.

If, after taking a break, you continue to have pain or numbness, you need to see your doctor or sports medicine consultant. Nerve pain is serious and needs to be addressed before big or irreversible problems occur.

## Back Pain

Back pain is one of the more common complaints in cycling. Like many of the problems discussed here, back pain is often position related. This may include position on the bike, position at work, and position when you stand. In general, many people have chronic bad posture, and this places undue strain on the lower-back skeleton and muscles.

Once back pain develops, you may need to see a health care professional to evaluate the problem and determine the source of the problem. Are your muscles in balance? Either your hamstring muscles or quadriceps muscles may be disproportionately strong compared to the other. Isolation strength exercises, such as leg extension and leg curl, can help equalize the pull on your back. Much of this should be done in the off-season, but it is never too late to try to improve your back health. You may want to work with a trainer or physical therapist who can show you proper strengthening technique.

Do you have a disc problem? Over time, undue pressure and strain are placed on your intervertebral discs, causing the disc to bulge or even rupture. This is a serious problem and sometimes needs intervention and surgery. Don't let your problem get to this point.

Work on having good back posture. This applies to all aspects of your life, not just cycling. If you sit at work, maintain good posture and get yourself a good chair. Make sure you get up and walk around periodically to avoid tightening of your muscles. If you have to pick up items or do manual work, always use good mechanics. Remember to use your legs and avoid bending at the back to pick items up.

## Hip Pain (Piriformis)

This problem is usually the result of muscle tightness and imbalance. The piriformis is a small muscle that helps rotate your leg outward. Much of the pedaling strength comes from the gluteus maximus. The piriformis, on the other hand, gets a free ride. This causes it to weaken and sometimes shorten. As a result, you get muscle tightness and pain.

The solution is a common theme—balance your muscles. This can be done in the gym by performing simple varied exercises. Perform complete range-of-motion workouts that include abduction and adduction exercises. You will also need to stretch and lengthen the piriformis.

Here's one useful exercise: Lie on your back, bend your knees, and place your right ankle on your left knee. Now, pull your left leg toward your trunk (figure 15.1a). You should feel the pull along the outside of your buttock. You can also increase the stretch by holding the same position while sitting on a foam roller (figure 15.1b). As you hold the position, slowly roll your buttock back and forth over the roller.

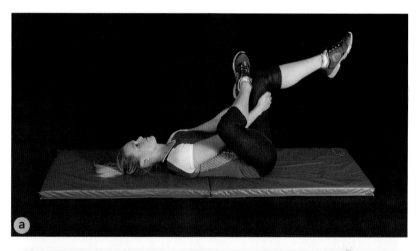

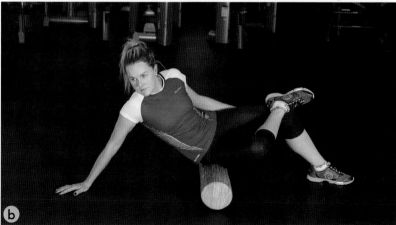

**Figure 15.1** *(a)* Hip stretch; *(b)* hip stretch with roller.

# Knee Pain

Knee pain is among the most common problems encountered by cyclists. For cyclists, the two main culprits of knee pain are position and overuse.

As discussed in chapter 14, a few of the parameters that determine your bike fit involve the knee. Obviously, saddle height plays a big role. Remember, anytime you change a shoe or cleat, you will have to reevaluate your saddle height. The second fit parameter is your cleat position on the shoe. This includes both the rotation of the foot and the fore-aft position. Both of these can cause knee pain if not properly aligned.

If you develop pain, you'll need to rest. While you're taking a break, think about your position and if you've had any changes recently. Have you ramped up your miles? You may need to visit a local bike fit company to ensure that you have good mechanics and position.

A problem that is often overlooked is cleat position. Your setup should put you in a neutral position with regard to your foot pedal position. Neutral doesn't mean straight along the axis of the frame. Neutral represents your natural position. Look down when you are just standing. Are you pigeon-toed, straight, or duck-footed? Your foot position should look similar when you are sitting on your bike at rest with your foot in the forward, crank-up position (3 or 9 o'clock depending on the foot).

I hate to admit it, but when I started to age, I developed some knee pain. I switched to a free-floating pedal system (Speedplay), and my knee problems went away.

Kneecap pain can arise from patellofemoral pain syndrome or chondro-malacia. These are fancy terms for overuse injury and wear and tear on the body. The track below the kneecap becomes inflamed from the movement of the knee during pedaling. This can be accelerated by degenerating carti-lage due to age and use. The solution is rest and good alignment. You may need to strengthen various aspects of your quadriceps muscle. Remember, the muscle consists of four parts, and if any head becomes out of balance, your kneecap may not track well in its groove.

Stretching can also help alleviate knee pain. Again, you may have a muscle balance or length issue, and stretching will help resolve the issue.

# Foot Issues

Foot issues essentially come down to finding a shoe that is compatible with your particular foot shape. Everybody's foot is shaped differently, and each shoe manufacturer has different features that work well for some and not others. For example, one maker's products are better for wider feet, whereas another's products are better for thin feet. I've been with riders who were required to wear poor fitting shoes because of sponsorship obligations.

They've gone to the extreme of cutting small holes over their little toes to stop the chaffing and irritation.

Fortunately for you, you only have to worry about comfort and fit. Get a shoe based not on brand, but on best fit. Your shoe should be snug but not too tight. It should let your foot breathe and swell in the heat.

If you develop an area of pain due to constant rubbing against the shoe, try to stretch that area of the plastic or leather with direct pressure. You can also use a cutout foam "donut" to place over the inflamed site. If you don't address the problem, things will only get worse. The constant pressure will result in your body responding with inflammation. This in turn causes bone and tissue to grow in the area of contact. A vicious circle ensues—more inflammation causing more growth causing more inflammation.

The solution is a properly fitting shoe. Try numerous pairs to find the best fit. Don't sacrifice your riding because you happen to have accidently picked up a bad pair of shoes. As mentioned previously, you shouldn't skimp on items for the areas of contact with your bike. Your saddle and shoes are your primary interface with the bike.


Make sure you always take care of yourself. It doesn't pay to be a hero with your training. Be sensible and address problems early. Remember to always ease into your training. The same is true of new equipment, such as shoes and shorts, or adjustments to your position. Stay on track for the long haul. The goal is to progress from season to season; impatience can lead to long-standing complications. If you train smart and pay attention to the messages your body gives you, you should be able to keep your progression moving in the right direction.

# Appendix A

## Personal Training Zones

## Intensity Levels Based on LTHR

| | % of LTHR | | Your LTHR |
|---|---|---|---|
| **Zone 1: Active recovery** | High end of zone | <80% | <.80 × _____ = |
| **Zone 2: Endurance** | Low end of zone | 80% | .80 × _____ = |
| | High end of zone | 90% | .90 × _____ = |
| **Zone 3: Tempo** | Low end of zone | 90% | .90 × _____ = |
| | High end of zone | 97% | .97 × _____ = |
| **Zone 4: Lactate threshold** | Low end of zone | 97% | .97 × _____ = |
| | High end of zone | 103% | 1.03 × _____ = |
| **Zone 5: Super threshold** | Low end of zone | 103% | 1.03 × _____ = |
| | High end of zone | 110% | 1.10 × _____ = |
| **Zone 6: Maximal** | Low end of zone | >109% | >1.10 × _____ = |

## Intensity Levels Based on LT Power

| | % of LT power | | Your LT power |
|---|---|---|---|
| **Zone 1: Active recovery** | High end of zone | <50% | <.50 × _____ = |
| **Zone 2: Endurance** | Low end of zone | 50% | .50 × _____ = |
| | High end of zone | 75% | .75 × _____ = |
| **Zone 3: Tempo** | Low end of zone | 75% | .75 × _____ = |
| | High end of zone | 99% | .99 × _____ = |
| **Zone 4: Lactate threshold** | High end of zone | 100% | 1.00 × _____ = |
| **Zone 5: Super threshold** | Low end of zone | 100% | 1.00 × _____ = |
| | High end of zone | 150% | 1.50 × _____ = |
| **Zone 6: Maximal** | Low end of zone | >150% | 1.50 × _____ = |

 From S. Sovndal, 2013, *Fitness cycling* (Champaign, IL: Human Kinetics).

## Intensity Levels Based on MHR

| | % of MHR | | Your MHR |
|---|---|---|---|
| **Zone 1: Active recovery** | High end of zone | <60% | <.60 × _____ = |
| **Zone 2: Endurance** | Low end of zone | 60% | .60 × _____ = |
| | High end of zone | 72% | .72 × _____ = |
| **Zone 3: Tempo** | Low end of zone | 72% | .72 × _____ = |
| | High end of zone | 79% | .79 × _____ = |
| **Zone 4: Lactate threshold** | Low end of zone | 80% | .80 × _____ = |
| | High end of zone | 90% | .90 × _____ = |
| **Zone 5: Super threshold** | Low end of zone | 91% | .91 × _____ = |
| | High end of zone | 97% | .97 × _____ = |
| **Zone 6: Maximal** | Low end of zone | >98% | .98 × _____ = |

# Appendix B

## Training Logs

# Simple Training Diary Log

Date _____

Ride description _____

Distance _____

Time _____

Intensity _____

Emotional state (happy, sad, distracted, stressed) _____

_____

Sleep _____

Fatigue level _____

Fitness level _____

# Advanced Training Diary Log

Date _____

Ride description _____

Distance _____

Time _____

Intensity _____

Emotional state (happy, sad, distracted, stressed) _____

_____

Sleep _____

Fatigue level _____

Fitness level _____

Average speed _____

Average cadence _____

Average power _____

Maximum heart rate _____

Average heart rate _____

Time in heart rate zones _____

Maximum power _____

Average power _____

Total work (in kilojoules/calories) _____

From S. Sovndal, 2013, *Fitness cycling* (Champaign, IL: Human Kinetics).

## Create Your Own Program

| Week | Mon | Tues | Wed | Thurs | Fri | Sat | Sun |
|------|-----|------|-----|-------|-----|-----|-----|
| 1 | | | | | | | |
| 2 | | | | | | | |
| 3 | | | | | | | |
| 4 | | | | | | | |
| 5 | | | | | | | |
| 6 | | | | | | | |

From S. Sovndal, 2013, *Fitness cycling* (Champaign, IL: Human Kinetics).

# Index

# About the Author

**Shannon Sovndal, MD,** is the team physician for the Garmin-Sharp-Barracuda professional cycling team and works at the General Clinical Research Center (GCRC) for the University of Colorado. He attended medical school at Columbia University in New York City and completed his residency at Stanford University. He is a member of the American College of Sports Medicine and the American College of Emergency Medicine.

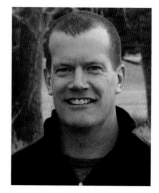

Before becoming a physician, Sovndal raced road bikes in the United States, winning the California/Nevada District Championship and numerous other road races and criteriums. He has written several articles on cycling topics and contributed to the scientific literature in emergency medicine. He coauthored the previous version of *Fitness Cycling* and was lead author of *Cycling Anatomy*, both published by Human Kinetics.